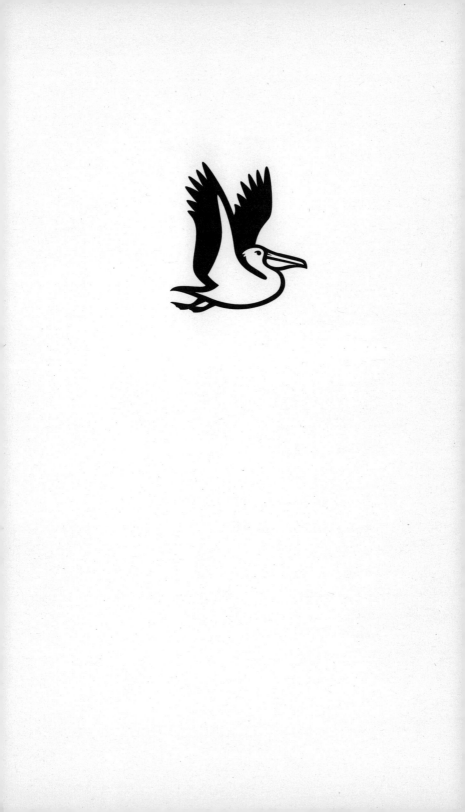

RICHARD LAYARD
WITH GEORGE WARD

Can We Be Happier?
Evidence and Ethics

A PELICAN BOOK

PELICAN
an imprint of
PENGUIN BOOKS

PELICAN BOOKS

UK | USA | Canada | Ireland | Australia
India | New Zealand | South Africa

Penguin Books is part of the Penguin Random
House group of companies whose addresses can
be found at global.penguinrandomhouse.com.

 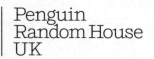

Penguin
Random House
UK

First published 2020
001

Text copyright © Richard Layard and George Ward, 2020

The moral right of the author has been asserted

Book design by Matthew Young
Set in 11/16.13 pt FreightText Pro
Typeset by Jouve (UK), Milton Keynes
Printed and bound in Great Britain by
Clays Ltd, Elcograf S.p.A.

A CIP catalogue record for this book is available
from the British Library

ISBN: 978–0–241–42999–0

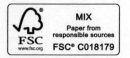

Penguin Random House is committed to a
sustainable future for our business, our readers
and our planet. This book is made from Forest
Stewardship Council® certified paper.

www.greenpenguin.co.uk

To the Dalai Lama
for the inspiration you give us
and to Molly
for our wonderful love

Contents

The Two Cultures

> Whoever is happy will make others happy too . . . How
> wonderful it is that nobody need wait a single moment
> before starting to improve the world.
> — Anne Frank, *The Diary of a Young Girl*

There is a wind of change in our society. People are talking about feelings. Even men are doing it. Quite recently Prince William and Prince Harry talked for the first time about their mother's death and how it affected their own mental health. There is a new undercurrent of concern with our own inner life and with how other people feel. Despite appearances, a new gentler culture is emerging.

By contrast, the older culture, which still dominates, is altogether harsher. It is more focused on externals. It encourages people to aim above all at personal success: good grades, a good job, a good income and a desirable partner. This culture of striving has brought many blessings, and life today is probably as good as it has ever been in human history. But that culture also involves a lot of stress, and people wonder why – if we are now so much richer than previous generations – we are not a lot happier?

The answer is surely the ultra-competitive nature of the dominant culture. The objective it offers is success compared with other people. But, if I succeed, someone else has to fail. So we have set ourselves up for a zero-sum game: however hard we all try to succeed, there can be no increase in overall happiness. An alternative, gentler culture offers a different aim, which can lead to a win–win outcome. It says that we should of course take care of ourselves, but we should get as much happiness as possible from contributing to the happiness of others.

Competition, it argues, is valuable in the right context – and that context is competition between organizations. This has been a major engine of progress. But what we need between individuals is mostly cooperation, not competition.[1] We want people who will act for the greater good – at work, at home and in the community. This produces better results for everyone. But, above all, it makes life more enjoyable. For people long to relate well to each other – as an end in itself and not just as a means to something else.

So the basic proposal in this book is that we should each of us, in all our choices, aim to produce the greatest happiness that we can – and especially the least misery. This noble vision does not go against basic human nature. For all of us have two inherited traits – one selfish and one altruistic. The selfish side believes that I am the centre of the universe and my needs come first. This trait was important for our survival as a race, and we should indeed take good care of ourselves and of our own inner equilibrium.

But the altruistic side enables us to feel what others feel and to strive for their good. This is vital for a happy society. It is a fallacy to think that reputation is a sufficient motivation for good behaviour. We need people with an inner desire to live good lives, even without reward. A happy society requires a lot of altruism, and so it needs a culture which supports our altruistic side.[2]

This gentler culture has always been around, in some form or other. It is there in all the great religions. Yet for many people these religions have lost their ability to convince. As religious belief has declined, a void has been created and into that void has rushed egotism, by default. We have told our young people that their chief duty is to themselves – to get on. What a terrible responsibility. No wonder that anxiety and depression are rising amongst the young.[3] Instead, people need to get out of themselves – to escape the misery of self-absorption. So there has to be a new, secular ethic, based on human need and not divine command.

The political crisis

A secular ethic is also vital if our democracies are to thrive. There is massive discontent with the world's elite, and with the atomistic neo-liberalism which it often espouses. According to that philosophy, all will go well if individuals are free to negotiate their own way through life; selfishness is not a problem provided people can choose their own friends and trading partners. But this ignores one key fact – that we would all be better off if the pool of possible friends and traders were nicer and more honest. For all of us the attitude of other people is crucial.

For this reason there is now a strong push back against extreme liberalism. People are calling for a society based on 'reciprocal obligation'.[4] In this view, we do not enter this world as independent, fully fledged adults, but as people highly dependent on support from our family, our government and the whole of our society. In return for this, we should ourselves feel bound to help others when we can. We want a free society, but one where people feel a duty to help.

But help in what way? There needs to be a clear content to our obligation to others. I think this is best expressed in terms of happiness: our obligation is to create the most happiness that we can in the society around us. This is the ideology we need for the twenty-first century. It is the vision of society that politicians should champion, and it is the principle that should guide their priorities in government. It is also, as we shall see, the principle that will get them re-elected. So the aim of politicians, as of private individuals, should be to create as much happiness in the world as possible and as little misery.

The happiness revolution

This new secular ethics is the basic principle for the happiness revolution – for both individuals and governments. But to implement it we have to know what makes people happy – both other people and ourselves. Two major developments now make this more possible. One is the new 'science of happiness' which gives policy-makers new knowledge about how to improve happiness and reduce misery. And the other is the new psychology of 'mind-training' which enables us all to get a better control over our own inner mental life. So, as Figure 0.1 shows, there are altogether three elements behind the amazing change that is now under way in our society.

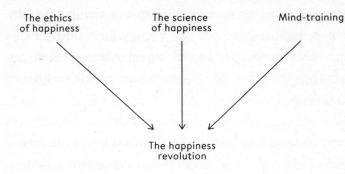

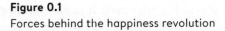

Figure 0.1
Forces behind the happiness revolution

Let us look briefly at each of these elements. The basic **secular ethics** goes back to the eighteenth-century Anglo-Scottish Enlightenment, which proposed a radically new goal for society. The goal, it said, should be the happiness of the people. That Happiness Principle was, I believe, the most important idea of the modern age, with powerful implications for how we should live and how our policy-makers should act on our behalf.

According to this principle, each of us should aim to create the most happiness in the world that we can and the least misery. And policy-makers and governments likewise should aim at the greatest happiness of the people and the least misery. This principle inspired many of the great social reforms of the nineteenth century, but it was soon challenged by philosophies that glorified struggle. Such dreadful philosophies contributed to two world wars and to the ultra-competitive features of today's dominant culture.

But now the Happiness Principle is making a comeback.

There are many reasons for this. One is disillusion with the dominant culture and the stress which people experience at every level of society. But the other reasons are hugely positive. Now, for the first time, we have a **science of happiness**, which gives us real evidence on how to create a happier society. This is relevant to all of us, but it also gives policy-makers new insights into the main causes of misery – and a new understanding of deprivation and how to address it.

At the same time there are new techniques of **mind-training** that enable each of us to improve our own inner mental state. The story began in the 1970s with breakthroughs in the psychological treatment of mental distress, based on scientifically controlled trials. Following on from that has come positive psychology, with evidence-based ways in which all of us can become happier. And, finally, more and more people now use age-old Eastern meditation to achieve greater contentment and calm of mind.

In Chapters 1–3 of the book we discuss each of the three strands in our diagram (see Figure 0.1). They all have one common element – they focus on the inner life as the ultimate reality for every human being. And they offer the prospect of a society where we take care, more than ever, of our own inner contentment and, especially, the happiness of others.

But does this new culture have any chance of replacing the dominant culture? For many people it has already done so. For them this new way of thinking is already fully established: they are members of a growing world happiness movement. These people include:

- millions who use meditation, mindfulness, yoga, positive psychology and other practices that support a contented way of living
- workers in mental health care, counselling and coaching – one of the most rapidly growing professions
- many of their beneficiaries, as well as people using self-help, Alcoholics Anonymous and so on
- educators teaching the skills of living, from primary schools to top universities
- thousands of companies and managers who care about the wellbeing of their workers and not just their performance
- policy-makers worldwide who fight for policies based on human values rather than the maximization of GDP, and
- researchers who provide the evidence-base for these policies.

This movement is affecting people in all walks of life – from rich to poor and from the happiest to those in despair.

Here are some graphs which illustrate the change (see Figure 0.2). The first two are from the media. If we look at *The Guardian* newspaper, the percentage of articles including 'happiness' has doubled since 2010 and the percentage including 'mental health' has risen by a factor of five. There is also a huge increase in the amount of published peer-reviewed research on happiness. From virtually nothing in 2000, this has reached nearly 2,000 articles a year. Even in economics journals there are already 200 articles a year on the subject.

And finally there are the changes in lifestyle. In the USA 14 per cent of all adults report that they have meditated in the past twelve months, and 17 per cent have been to a yoga class.[5] Nearly 50 per cent live in households where someone has visited a mental-health professional in the last year.[6] All these activities are growing rapidly and the final graph shows the hugely increased interest in both meditation and yoga. I am often amazed when talking to a cabinet minister, top official or top businessman to find they have been meditating for years – in secret, of course.

But let's be honest. Even though interest in it has blossomed, this is still a minority culture and in the final chapter of Part One I will discuss the cross-winds that are blowing in the opposite direction. To overcome these cross-winds will require huge effort and clarity of purpose from all of us.

What can each of us do?

So how can we each become more effective as creators of happiness, both as citizens and in our own occupation, whatever that is? These are the issues we address in Part Two of the book:

- How can we as individuals find more happiness and contribute better to the happiness of others?
- How can teachers help children to become creators of happiness?
- How can managers make work more enjoyable?
- How can health-workers heal our minds as well as our bodies?
- How can couples find happiness and bring up happy children?

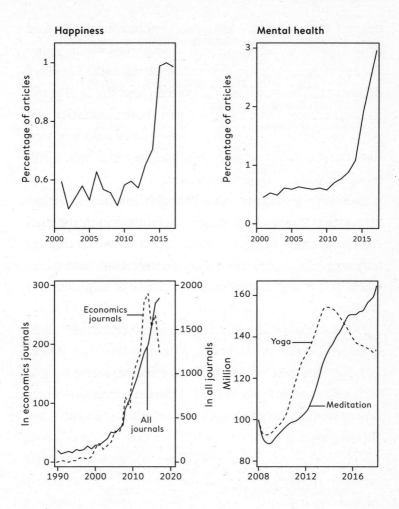

Figure 0.2

(*top*) Articles in *The Guardian* newspaper mentioning happiness and mental health
(*bottom left*) Articles on happiness in academic journals
(*bottom right*) Google searches for meditation and yoga

- How can local communities provide the social and physical basis for happy living?
- How can economists like myself provide good policy advice, aimed at happiness?
- How can politicians create happier societies?
- What are the priorities for science and technology, if happiness is the aim?

To answer these questions I draw on the vast mass of evidence now emerging on what works best for happiness. Wherever possible, the evidence I present comes from properly controlled experiments. The experimental method has been well established in medicine for over a century, but more recently it has spread into social science.[7] And happiness is increasingly included as a measured outcome – in my opinion it is the most important one. So this book reports cutting-edge science, directed at human happiness.

This is an extraordinarily exciting time. Cultural change can be quite rapid if the right idea arises at the right time.[8] The Happiness Principle is an idea whose time has come. Most people now realize that economic growth, however desirable, will not solve all our problems. Instead we need a philosophy and a science which encompasses a much fuller range of human experience.

The growing influence of women in society is helping this revolution. Research suggests that most women care more about inner feelings than men do, while typically men focus more on external issues.[9] Moreover, women are typically more altruistic than men, and more concerned with how others feel, and so their increasing power and influence will help to ensure that the happiness movement succeeds.[10]

For all these reasons, I am confident that this surging, subterranean movement will eventually become mainstream and displace the dominant culture of today.

My own involvement

We all have our part to play in this happiness revolution. But how, you might ask, did I, as an economist of all things, become involved in it? It is actually not surprising. Economics was originally founded in order to discover which institutions would produce the greatest happiness for the people. As soon as I discovered this, I switched to economics. As I explain in my thanks at the end of the book, I was by that time in my thirties. However, I was quickly shocked by the narrow view economists had about what actually causes happiness. Essentially they thought it was about purchasing power, plus a few other bits and pieces.

The fallacy of this assumption was already apparent by 1974 when Richard Easterlin showed that US citizens were getting no happier despite the country's rapid economic growth. I thought then of writing a book about happiness, but instead I wrote an article.[11] For at that time there was little research evidence on what makes people happy. But by 1998 there was much more, and we invited Daniel Kahneman, the psychologist who subsequently won the Nobel Prize in Economics, over to London to lecture on the new science of happiness. Soon after that I decided to write my own book on Happiness. I rang Kahneman for advice and he replied, 'First read the collected essays on Wellbeing that I've just published and then come to Princeton.' I did, and it was one of the most exciting times of my life. I also visited the founder of positive psychology, Martin Seligman, and the laboratory of Richard Davidson, where he carried out his ground-breaking work on the neuroscience of happiness.

The next thing was an email from a Buddhist monk in Nepal. Richard Davidson had written to his Buddhist friend Matthieu Ricard about this British economist who was working on happiness. In due course, Matthieu arrived at our house in his red and saffron robes, and I became aware of the wonderful Mind and Life group of Western scholars who meet regularly with the Dalai Lama to discuss the relation between Buddhist and Western psychology. Through this group I came to know the Dalai Lama, who has probably done more than any living person to advance the cause of happiness.

So I have met many inspiring people and had many unexpected experiences. Perhaps the strangest of all was organizing courses on mindfulness for British Members of Parliament. They lapped it up. Some MPs even said their lives had been changed forever.

After I had finished writing *Happiness*, I asked myself, What can I do next which will help to reduce misery? I concluded that the area of mental health was where I could do the most. But how? In 2003 I had become a Fellow of the British Academy and duly went to a very stiff inaugural tea party. I was standing next to a tall, good-looking chap and asked him what he did. He turned out to be David Clark, one of the world's leading clinical psychologists. I have worked with him ever since.

In 2004 it was virtually impossible for people with depression or crippling anxiety disorders to get psychological therapy in Britain's National Health Service. So David and I made the case for a completely new service. He provided the technical expertise; I provided the economic argument and the political connections. Tony Blair had made me a Labour Party member of the House of Lords, and so we were able to present our case to a seminar at 10 Downing Street. Eventually, after many more meetings, the case was accepted. Thanks to David's leadership the service now treats over half a million sufferers a year, half of whom recover during a course of treatment. The service is so successful that it is now being copied in at least five other countries.

But happiness is more than mental health. If the Happiness Principle and all it implies is to become embedded in our culture, it needs an organization to promote it. Every successful culture has institutions that enshrine its principles. Religious cultures have churches, temples, synagogues or mosques. But where is the organization that is dedicated to the Greatest Happiness Principle, and where do its followers meet regularly to be inspired and supported in living good lives? That was the next challenge.

In 2006 I was in a TV debate with Anthony Seldon, the newly appointed head of a private secondary school called Wellington College. He had just introduced happiness lessons into the school, despite considerable scepticism from teachers and school governors. We had an immediate rapport and soon we got together with Geoff Mulgan, the former head of Tony Blair's policy unit, and decided to launch a movement that could fill the organizational gap. Its aim is to inspire individuals to live good, happy lives – through its website and even more through face-to-face groups that meet regularly to inspire and to be inspired.

We called the movement Action for Happiness. It attracted good candidates for the post of director, including one who prior to the interview had Googled the question 'What organizations have the word "happiness" in their titles?' The search engine's reply was 'Your search for happiness has produced no results.' That was 2011. Things have changed since then. Thanks to its great director, Mark Williamson, Action for Happiness now has over a million online followers and 150,000 members in 180 countries.

Finally, there is the global policy challenge: to persuade policy-makers to make happiness their goal. In 2004 the Organization for Economic Cooperation and Development (OECD), the club of rich countries, held the first of many conferences on the subject of 'What is Progress?' The next step was to get countries to measure the happiness of their people as part of their routine national gathering of statistics. Fortunately, Britain's Cabinet Secretary Gus O'Donnell was on side and in 2011 Britain became the first country to do that. At the same time, one of the world's leading development economists, Jeffrey Sachs (who was also adviser to the UN Secretary General), became a strong advocate for happiness. Since then, he, John Helliwell and I have edited the annual World Happiness Report, and more and more governments are now moving towards happiness as the goal of policy.

This book

But, even so, many in the world today (including many of my own friends) are barely aware of the world happiness movement and the way it is challenging many of the worst features of the dominant individualistic culture. This book tries to remedy that ignorance – and then to lay out how members of the happiness movement can in practice transform the lives of those they touch.

This book has two parts. Part One describes the ideas, science and behaviours which are generating the happiness revolution and the world happiness movement. This section is mainly directed at people who are not yet on board and need to be persuaded. By contrast, Part Two is directed at people who are already on board and want a happier world. It offers scientific evidence to show how each of us, in our own sphere of life, can contribute to bringing that about.

The book cannot possibly cover everything that needs doing. It focuses mainly on those key areas that are at the top of the new happiness agenda.[12] And it constantly stresses that this is not an expensive exercise. Most of the things that can be done are immensely cost-effective and, in many cases, pay for themselves. They are not luxury expenditures. They are critical for the happiness of billions, and they cost peanuts compared with much of what is spent to promote economic growth.

So let's put people first and mean it. We have enough knowledge – let's put it into action. The world happiness movement will surely go from strength to strength. What is counter-cultural today will in time become the mainstream. And the result will be a happier society.

PART ONE

The Happiness Revolution

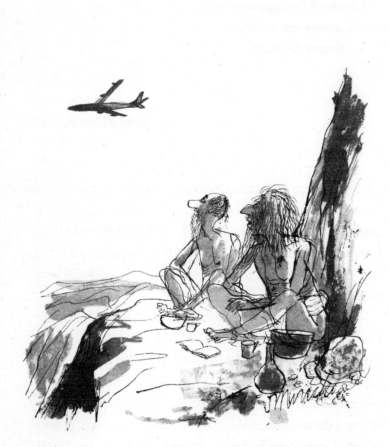

"They have the know-how, but do they have the know-why?"

What's the Purpose?

> Create all the happiness you are able to create: remove all
> the misery you are able to remove.
> — Jeremy Bentham[1]

A few years ago I was asked to give a lunchtime talk at Goldman Sachs's offices in London. Until then the record attendance at these talks had been 500, to hear the tennis star Martina Navratilova. There were 810 in the audience for my talk – not because of me, but because of the title: 'Can we be happier?'

I believe passionately that we can and should have a happier way of life, and that the new science of happiness can help us towards it. In this book I try to show how it could happen: what we can each do as individuals, plus the huge potential contributions from teachers, managers, therapists, parents, economists, scientists and policy-makers in general. We shall look at each of these groups in turn.

But first we need to look more closely at the goal. Is greater happiness really the right goal for our society? Or should we just have lots of goals? The problem with multiple goals is what to do when one goal conflicts with another – when, for example, the redistribution of income conflicts with personal freedom. So in practice we have to have one over-arching goal. But what should it be?

Everyone wants to be happy. And most people want others to be happy also – at the very least they want it for their family and friends. We also have other wants, which are quite specific – for income, health, freedom, appreciation, friendship and so on. But if we ask why these other things matter to us, we can always give some reason – for example that they will make us feel better. On the other hand, if we ask why it matters that people feel happier, we can give no further answer. Happiness is self-evidently good, and one can convincingly argue that other goods derive their value from the way in which they contribute to our happiness. So happiness is the overarching good.[2]

But whose happiness? I obviously feel that my happiness matters, but everyone else feels the same about theirs. So it is impossible to argue that any one person's happiness is ultimately more important than anyone else's. It follows that the goal for a society must be the greatest possible happiness all round. Inevitably some people will be happier than others, but (as I shall argue later) we should take special care to raise up those with the lowest levels of happiness.[3] Subject to that qualification, the goal for any society should be the happiness of the people.

So how should each of us live our lives? Unfortunately some people think there is no such thing as 'should'. But if you believe there is such a thing, then we *should* obviously try to produce the best possible state of society around us – in other words, the greatest possible happiness that we can.

The Happiness Principle

Thus the starting point for this book is three key ideas which should, I believe, be central to a civilized society.

THE PROGRESS PRINCIPLE

We should judge the state of the world by how far people are enjoying their lives – by the amount of happiness there is, especially among those who are least happy. That, rather than GDP, should be our measure of progress. And, crucially, everybody's happiness matters equally.[4]

Next, turning to individuals, our duty must be to promote the best possible state of the world, in whatever way we can – which leads to the next idea.

THE ETHICAL PRINCIPLE

Each of us should aim, in the way we live and in the choices we make, to create the most happiness we can in the world around us, especially among those who are least happy.

This should be the key principle of moral philosophy. Morality, it says, is not just about avoiding bad behaviour: it is about positively promoting the good of others – in other words their happiness. This is an uplifting message which can inspire everyone in their daily lives, and should become second nature to young children as early as possible. Only a clear message like this can save us from self-absorption. But it is not a hair-shirt philosophy – it calls for joyful living, where we care for others but also for ourselves.

Finally there is the goal for the policy-makers who act

on our behalf either in government or in non-government organizations (NGOs). What should this be?

THE POLICY PRINCIPLE

Policy-makers should choose policies which create the greatest possible happiness, especially among those who are least happy.

This should be the central idea of political philosophy. If people are looking for a definition of the common good, this is it: the happiness of the people.

Some history

Taken together, these ideas comprise the Happiness Principle. None of them are new. In the form I have described them, they go back to the great eighteenth-century Anglo-Scottish Enlightenment. The Enlightenment replaced the idea that morality comes from God with the idea that our duty comes from our membership of society. Happiness was no longer postponed to the afterlife, but was to be promoted here and now. This was the defining idea of the modern age.[5]

However, unfortunately there remained in Western culture a strong streak of Puritanism. Many, even among the irreligious, felt that happiness was not enough. In their view, what made sense of life was struggle itself, rather than the fruits of struggle. This philosophy, epitomized by the Social Darwinists and Nietzsche, was strongest on the European continent. But even elsewhere there were many who justified the causes they fought for by something other than improvements in the quality of individual lives.[6] Many of the disasters of the twentieth century were influenced by this belief in the intrinsic merits of struggle.

Fortunately, since the Second World War, life has been better and is probably on average as good as in any previous period. But false gods still dominate much of our thinking. The most obvious is the idea that the only good is GDP – in other words that people exist to produce output, rather than output existing to serve the people. GDP has its value of course, but it is only one of many things that contribute to the overarching good, which is happiness.

Even so, is greater happiness really the best alternative goal for society? Three obvious questions arise.

Is happiness a serious enough objective?

Happiness means feeling good. But many people argue that happiness is a transient state: you cannot always be happy, so we need a more solid goal. But this is a misconception of what is being advocated. There are not two states, happy and un-happy, any more than there are two states, rich and poor. There is a scale of happiness, from very happy at the top to desper-ately miserable at the bottom – just as there is a scale of income from rich to poor. Moreover, people's levels of happiness fluc-tuate, and what we are concerned with here is their underlying happiness, averaged over a long period of time – how their life feels to them. What we want to see is happier lives.

So we are using the word happiness in exactly the same way that it is used in common parlance. For example, people may ask: how happy is your child at school? Or, how happy are you in your job? Or, are you happily married? Everyone knows what these questions mean: they are trying to find out how you feel about that aspect of your life.

We are just going one step further and asking, how good

do you feel about your whole life these days? Nobody can be happy all the time. In fact, if you are trying to do something worthwhile you are almost bound to feel frustrated at frequent intervals. Moreover, work is often hard, as is running a marathon. We do not do everything we do because it will make us happy at the time. We do it because in general we will feel good about it.

Even so, many sensible people have difficulty with the idea of 'happiness' or 'feeling good' as the ultimate goal for society. Many people prefer the word 'wellbeing'. But when asked to define it they often struggle. This is not surprising since the word 'wellbeing' is not a part of ordinary English: there is no adjective to describe a person with good wellbeing. That is why I prefer the word 'happiness' – people know what it means to be happy. But for most purposes either word will do.

So how can we best measure it? The most frequently used concept, by academics and policy-makers alike, is overall life-satisfaction. People are asked: 'Overall, how satisfied are you with your life these days', on a scale of 0–10 with 0 indicating 'Not at all satisfied' and 10 meaning 'Very satisfied'. The pattern of replies to the question remains very similar if the word 'happy' replaces the word 'satisfied'.[7]

Other specific questions about feelings can also be useful (especially when we are studying specific experiences over short periods of time). But, as an overall concept, I like the life-satisfaction, single-question approach rather than asking people lots of different questions and then weighting them into a single index – because then the researchers are forced to supply weights for each question rather than leaving it to individuals to make their own overall assessment. And in any case the weights differ between individuals. So life-satisfaction is the most democratic measure, since it is the respondents who decide what is good for them – and not some politician, bureaucrat or scholar.

Moreover, life-satisfaction is the measure that policy-makers prefer. They are used to asking people how satisfied they are with public services, so why not ask them about their life as a whole? Life-satisfaction is therefore the measure we use most frequently in this book.[8] We call it 'happiness', but by all means think of it as 'wellbeing', or 'quality of life' if you (like many policy-makers) prefer to do so.[9]

Does the happiness goal make people selfish?

Does talking about happiness mean we are encouraging selfishness? The answer to this question is a resounding 'No'. For what we are talking about is the goal for society, not a goal we are proposing for each individual. Clearly no society is going to be happy if each individual seeks only his or her own happiness – we are all deeply affected by how other people behave. So suppose the issue is how Jane (see Figure 1.1) should behave. Our Ethical Principle says that she should take into account the effect of her behaviour on both her own happiness and on the happiness of others. When she decides what to do with her life, she should take into account both of these effects. She should not just aim to be happy herself but to be a generator of happiness for herself *and* others.

A libertarian might say it is enough for her to pursue her

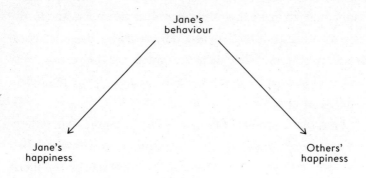

Figure 1.1
The effects of Jane's behaviour

own happiness, provided she does not reduce the happiness of others.[10] But no – as I have argued, she should actively seek to increase the happiness of others.

This highlights two different ways of looking at a society. The first is to ask how happy each person is. This is the standard procedure in studies of happiness. But, as we know, people's happiness depends hugely on how other people behave. So a second approach is to ask how each person is doing as a creator of happiness. This is surely equally important, since happiness can only be experienced if it is first created.

To see the difference between the two concepts, we can imagine a society consisting of only Jane and Emily. Jane is more giving than Emily, so she creates more happiness in Emily than Emily creates in her. Thus, overall, Jane creates more happiness than she herself experiences; and for Emily it is the other way around. This is illustrated in Figure 1.2. The first row shows how much happiness each of them

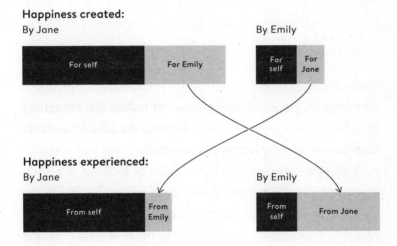

Happiness created:

By Jane

For self	For Emily

By Emily

For self	For Jane

Happiness experienced:

By Jane

From self	From Emily

By Emily

From self	From Jane

Figure 1.2
Happiness created and happiness experienced

creates. The second row shows how much happiness each experiences. Jane gives more happiness to Emily than she receives in return, so that she creates more happiness than she experiences. In the real world there are millions of people like Jane and millions of others like Emily, each of them affecting hundreds or thousands of other people.

This fundamental difference (between the happiness that a person experiences and the happiness which the same person creates) helps us to understand a long-standing controversy over the way we should measure happiness. The standard approach is to look at happiness experienced, through some measure like life-satisfaction. But others argue for something closer to what Aristotle had in mind when he talked about eudaemonia, which included a person's contribution to society. The natural measure of this is the happiness that person creates.[11]

Both approaches are of value. If we want to know who is suffering in a society and why, we certainly have to look at the happiness people experience. But if we want to build a happy society we need to know how to produce creators of happiness. When Aristotle talked of eudaemonia, he included virtue in the discussion. Virtue is of course difficult to measure but it is a key feature of the kind of citizens we would like to live with. Social scientists should therefore try to measure both happiness experienced, which is relatively easy, and happiness created.[12] For we will never understand the happiness and misery in our society unless we also study how people behave.

But how can we affect the way people behave? One approach is to appeal to their self-interest. People who behave well get treated better in return, so their reputation is a huge incentive to behave well. But that is not enough to create a truly happy society. We need people who behave well from habit not from calculation – people who help others, even if they will never see them again.

Such a society is quite possible. After all, people regularly help other people they will never see again, and they tolerate pain and discomfort doing things they think are right. Altruism is a daily reality.[13] So what makes it possible?

The answer seems to be a basic human mechanism whereby people feel happier if they are helping others – not all the time, but in general over their lives. There is good evidence that this is so – that altruistic behaviour makes people happier.[14] In one ingenious experiment Elizabeth Dunn divided a sample of students randomly into two groups. The first group were given money to spend on themselves, and the second group were given money to spend on other people. It turned out that spending money on others made the students happier than spending it on themselves. This experiment has been done in four very different countries with the same results. An equivalent experiment has also been performed on three-year-old toddlers, again with the same result: they smile more when they give away a treat than when they consume it themselves.

Similar results are found in real life. When Germany was reunited in 1990 the opportunities for volunteering in East Germany were drastically curtailed. The result was that East Germans who had previously volunteered became much less happy relative to other East Germans.[15] Equally, in careful comparisons between individuals, those who volunteer are on average happier and live longer.[16]

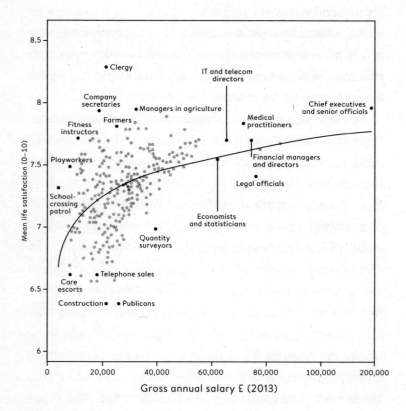

Figure 1.3
How occupations differ in average happiness and average salary in the UK

Because altruism matters so much, some people argue that virtue should be the ultimate aim of our society. But this is to confuse the means with the end. The end is a happy society, and virtue is a means to get there. So we are not offering a dismal philosophy where we constantly make ourselves miserable for the sake of others. We are promoting a generous spirit, where we get real meaning and enjoyment from what we do for others.

In the end, are we not simply restating Jesus's Golden Rule, 'Do to others what you want them to do to you'? That depends on what you want them to do to you. If you want them to make you happy, then yes, we are restating the Golden Rule. But if you want them to teach you the piano, that is probably not what they want of you. We should find out what makes them happy and do what we can to promote it.

The Happiness Principle applies to every choice we make in life: what to study, what job to take, how to manage our time and our family life, and what to do with our money. All morality is about the positive things we should do, as well as the negative ones we should avoid. For much of the unhappiness in the world is caused not by the bad things we do but by the good things we fail to do. Take, for example, the decision about what job to do. We should ask which choice will make the most difference to the happiness of others. What is it that we can do well and wouldn't happen unless we did it? And what will give us the most satisfaction ourselves?

So here, to whet your interest, is a graph showing the income and happiness people get from different occupations in Britain (see Figure 1.3). There is a big spread of both income and happiness, and there is some relation between the two. But the relation is not all that strong and there are huge differences between occupations paying the same money. So anyone wondering whether to enter an occupation is well advised to see how happy the people are who are already in that occupation. More details are in an online Annex.[17] But remember that these are only averages – you yourself might become happier or less happy than the average in that occupation. And of course you should also think about how that occupation affects the happiness of others.

What about social justice?

So far I have talked mainly as though the objective of society should be simply the total volume of happiness experienced in the society. In the eighteenth century this was Jeremy Bentham's approach. My approach would be different. I feel it is worse if A's life-satisfaction is 9 and B's is 5 than if both are at 7, even though the total is the same. That is my concept of social justice: I am concerned with how happiness is distributed. If you accept that happiness is the ultimate good, then social justice must be about how happiness is distributed between people.

In every society there is a wide spectrum of happiness – running from extreme misery to extreme happiness. The chart below shows the distribution of happiness in the British population (see Figure 1.4).[18] The least happy tenth obtain on average 3.8 points of happiness (out of a maximum possible of 10), and they are certainly in a lot of misery. By contrast, the most happy tenth obtain over 9 points out of 10. Some people are a lot luckier in their life than others.

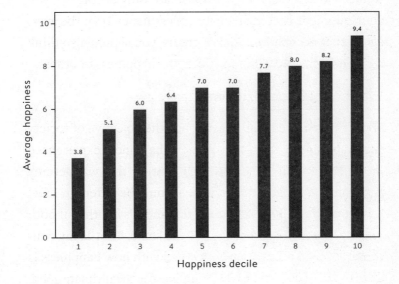

Figure 1.4
Average happiness of British people in each decile of happiness

	Before the policy change	After the policy change	Change in happiness
Most happy half	8	6	−2
Least happy half	4	5	+1
All	6	5.5	−0.5

Table 1.1
Average happiness (0–10) in each group

When judging a state of affairs, we need to take this spread of happiness into account, as well as simply the average level of happiness. We should be concerned in particular with the proportion of people in real misery. So if two societies have the same average happiness (as do, for example, Spain and Guatemala), but in one there is much more equality of happiness (as in Spain), then we prefer the situation in Spain. The difference between the countries is in fact huge, with 30 per cent of adults in Guatemala having happiness below 5 (out of 10) compared with only 15 per cent in Spain.[19]

Comparisons like that are simple, when average happiness is the same in both situations. But what if one situation provides greater average happiness, but is also more unequal? Let's take a practical example. Suppose a new policy has the following effect on the top and bottom half of the population. Average happiness in the population goes down, but the least happy people become happier (see Table 1.1).

Is this an improvement? It is the kind of choice that policy-makers face every day. And their decision depends on their values. The more egalitarian they are, the more weight they will give to the gain in happiness among those who are least happy. So what do you think?

Philosophers have a good thought-experiment for reflecting on this.[20] They ask, 'Suppose you were going to live in a society, but did not know which person you were going to be. In choosing between different situations, how much weight would you give to the average happiness in the society and how much to the inequality with which it was distributed?' In the present case which of the two situations shown would you prefer to be born into, if you did not know who you would be?

Everyone will have their own view. This is an area where personal values cannot be avoided, and we all have views on how much weight to give to increasing the happiness of the most miserable as compared to people higher up the scale.[21] But that is what defines the strength of our concern for social justice. The fundamental inequality in our society is the inequality of happiness, not of income.[22] Of course, one way to reduce misery is to reduce poverty, but as we shall see in the next chapter there are many others.

One important way to reduce misery is by establishing a set of legal rights, which rule out many kinds of bad outcomes. Such legal rights are a key part of any just society and flow naturally from the capabilities approach of my old friend and colleague Amartya Sen.[23]

But public policy should do more than secure a minimum of rights – it should help people of all kinds to live more fully, to flourish. For this purpose we need a clear overall objective: the happiness of the people.[24]

Conclusions

We need to replace the harsh culture in which we judge our lives by our success compared with others. That is a zero-sum game – the total of relative success can never be changed, however hard each person tries to improve their own position. Instead, we need a goal for each of us which can lead to progress for all. That goal has to be the positive-sum activity of contributing to a happier society.

If we want a happier society, we have to aim at it explicitly.

We will never achieve a happier society as a by-product. And it is a single overarching concept that we need if we are to displace the false idol of GDP. A dashboard of wellbeing indicators is certainly better than nothing, but it has been tried for half a century by the 'social indicators' movement with relatively little success. Rather, we need a single, clear concept that can inspire passion and effort because it corresponds to the basic wish of every human being – to feel good about her life.

So we need a new twenty-first-century Enlightenment which reclaims the basic eighteenth-century ideal, and where:

- we judge societies by their levels of happiness
- we try as individuals to create the most happiness we can and get as much of our own happiness as possible from increasing the happiness of others, and
- we expect our policy-makers to try to target the happiness of the people and especially to reduce the prevalence of misery.

To build this happier society is an ideal that can inspire us all, young and old. But do we have a chance of doing it? Is the goal feasible? I believe it is, and in this book I explain how we can take some first steps in this direction.

The rest of Part One looks at the main positive forces at work in our society, as well as some of the negative ones. By contrast, Part Two is addressed to one group after another, outlining how each can contribute to the building of a happier society. There can be no nobler task.

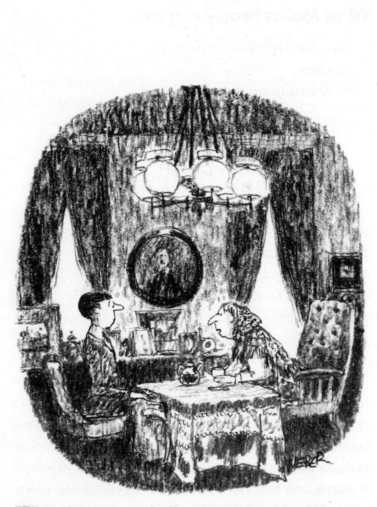

"*The tea leaves say you should go into insurance, but I say forget the tea leaves and go into whatever makes you happy.*"

What Makes People Happy?

> Everyone is entitled to his own opinion, but not to his
> own facts.
> — Senator Daniel Patrick Moynihan[1]

In the early 1980s Margaret Thatcher decided that wealth-creation should be the overarching aim of her government. At the same time a young assistant professor at the University of Illinois was moving in the opposite direction. He told his psychologist colleagues that he was going to study happiness. They said 'What nonsense', so the ingenious professor, named Ed Diener, said OK then, I'll work on 'subjective wellbeing'.

In the decades that followed, Diener and his psychological research group did literally hundreds of studies of the causes of happiness. They mainly studied the happiness of students, but also of people as different as the Maasai and the Inuit.[2] In due course, economists also became involved in happiness research, and they typically looked at larger populations. Richard Easterlin of the University of California, and then Andrew Oswald of the University of Warwick, spotted that questions about happiness had been asked in many general-purpose surveys of the whole population, with good sample sizes. These included the periodic World Values Surveys, as well as surveys which followed the same people year after year in Britain, Germany and Australia. Countless researchers have used these surveys to estimate how different factors affect a person's happiness.

But often these studies have focused on one cause at a time, making it difficult to compare the importance of different experiences in terms of their effect on happiness. So our research group at the London School of Economics has recently used all the main surveys to estimate these relationships in a way that makes it possible to compare the importance of each factor. This chapter is mainly based on our findings.[3]

Can happiness be measured?

But can we really compare the happiness of different people? Three things demonstrate that we can – at least to an approximation.

First, there is quite a good correlation between what people say and objective measurements taken from the brain. Richard Davidson has shown this not only in the same person (when their feelings are altered during an experiment) but also across individuals at rest. The neuroscience is still in its early days, but correlations such as these reinforce the view that people's self-reports have objective informational content.[4]

Second, what people say about their happiness turns out to have huge predictive power. It helps predict their productivity, and their chances of quitting their job or their marriage, and their length of life. A sample of people over fifty were given a medical examination, and they were also asked a set of questions about happiness. They were then followed for eight years to see how many of them died. It turned out that the

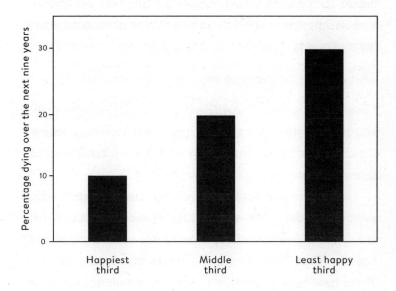

Figure 2.1
Happiness affects longevity (people originally aged fifty and over)

least happy third of people were 200 per cent more likely to die than the happiest third (see Figure 2.1).[5] Even when other influences were controlled for, the least happy people were still 50 per cent more likely to die than the happiest ones.

Finally, of course, there is the fact that we can to a good extent explain people's answers – why they differ in the happiness they report. And that is what this chapter is about. So how important are different factors in explaining who is happy and who is not?

The effects of income and unemployment

I have spent most of my life working on income inequality and unemployment. I thought they were the most important causes of unhappiness, but research on happiness has revealed a more complicated picture.

Unemployment is really tough, as I had thought, and on average it reduces life-satisfaction by about 0.7 points (out of 10) – similar to the effect of being widowed or separated.[6] But the effect of income is much less than I had expected. There have been thousands of surveys in hundreds of countries and they typically find that, holding all else constant, a person with double your income will be 0.2 points happier than you are. Similarly, a person whose income is one half of yours will be 0.2 points less happy.[7] These are not huge differences and in most countries income inequality explains under 2 per cent of the variance of happiness.[8]

However, the case for redistribution remains clear. For what matters to people is the proportional change in their income. So, suppose a poor person is receiving an extra $100, and this is coming from someone who is ten times richer. The poor person's gain in happiness will be ten times as large as the rich person's loss of happiness. Though the gain to the poor person may be less than you might have thought, it is still much greater than the loss to the rich person.

But an important issue still remains: could the rich person's dollar have been used to create even more happiness by some other policy than by giving it to someone who is poor? To answer this, we have to consider all the other causes of happiness. Which of them matter most?

What matters most?

To think about this, we can begin with the huge spread of life-satisfaction in the population which we saw on page 33 – ranging from misery to extreme happiness. We ask: what explains this variation? And to answer it we estimate an equation in which all the possible influences are included simultaneously. We can then calculate for each influence its 'partial correlation coefficient' with happiness. This measure, which we use frequently in the book, reflects how far each factor contributes independently to the overall variation of the thing being explained (in this case happiness).[9] The analysis in the following chart is for happiness in Britain, but the results in other industrialized countries are very similar.[10]

As can be seen from Figure 2.2, the main influences are to do with your health, physical and mental, and with your human relationships. The most striking influence is your mental health. But your family life and your life at work are also extremely important – which is not surprising when you consider how much of our time we spend at home or at work. Our genes are of course also important, but there is nothing

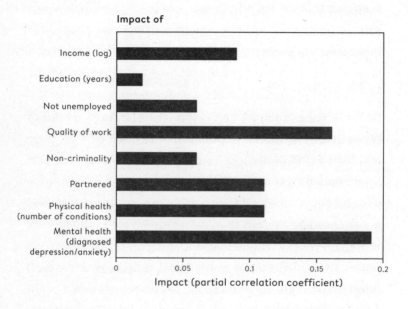

Figure 2.2
What explains the variation of adult happiness (in Britain)?

we can do about them.[11] On the other hand, we can do a lot about the other factors, with help from teachers, managers, health professionals and people who work with families and communities.

But, you might ask, do these findings underestimate the role of really low income as a key cause of distress? To investigate this we ask why some people have really low life-satisfaction, while others do not – why some people are miserable while others are not. This enables us to produce another figure like the one above, but one where we are explaining the presence or otherwise of misery (rather than the whole spread of happiness). For this purpose we measure misery by whether someone has a life-satisfaction score of less than 4 (out of 7).[12]

Remarkably, the new figure looks exactly like the figure above – the numbers are all slightly lower, but the pattern across the different factors is exactly the same.[13] Mental illness is the most important factor, followed by physical health and family life. Low income comes below these as a cause of misery. These are results for rich countries. In poorer countries, poverty is the most important factor, but even in poor countries mental illness is as important a cause of misery as physical illness is.[14]

A better concept of deprivation

So it is time we took the inner life more seriously. In fact, we clearly need a new definition of deprivation. A person is as deprived when they lack the inner means to enjoy life as when they lack the external means. At this point we have to confront a common misconception, popularized some seventy years ago by the psychologist Abraham Maslow.[15] He claimed there was a 'hierarchy of needs' beginning with the physical need for food, clothing and shelter, and reaching up through social needs to the need for spiritual exaltation. The idea of the hierarchy meant that, if your lower needs were unmet, there was no point thinking about your higher needs. Maslow provided no evidence for this and most of us have met people who are clearly flourishing with rich social connections and joy in their lives, but very little money. Empirical research confirms this.[16] If the happiness movement does nothing else, let's hope it can get rid of the hierarchy approach and convince people that mental health and a rich social life are as important to poor and rich alike.[17] And they matter as much in poor countries as in rich ones. Let 'Maslow' provide no excuse for the shocking neglect of mental health in poor countries.

So much for how our happiness as adults is affected by our life as adults. But didn't our childhood contribute to the adult we became? Which features of our childhood best predict our enjoyment of life as an adult?

What matters most in childhood?

There are three main aspects to how we develop as children: our academic achievement, our emotional health and our behaviour towards others. Which of these is the best predictor of whether we will have a happy adult life? In Britain it's not academic achievement. Our emotional development at sixteen is a better predictor of our adult happiness than the whole panoply of our educational qualifications, including degrees of all kinds.[18]

But what then determines a child's emotional health at age sixteen? Many people would think the child's parents would have the most influence on this. But a study in the English city of Bristol and its surroundings shows something quite remarkable. The study followed up all the children born in the area in 1991–2, and recorded which primary school and which secondary school they went to. Each of these schools had many children who were included in the study, so that it was possible to see what difference (on average) each school made to the emotional development of the children who went there. The difference was enormous.[19] In fact the happiness of a child at sixteen was equally affected by:

- which secondary school they were at;
- which primary school they had been to, and
- everything we know about their parents (their income, mental health, parenting skills, family conflict, etc.).

These results, discussed further in Chapter 6, show just how much difference teachers and parents can make to the happiness of their children – both when the children are young *and* when they have become adults.

So we can learn a lot by studying the differences between individuals in a given country. These differences within countries explain 80 per cent of the variation in happiness across the whole human race.[20] So there is no reason why you should not be happy just because of where you live – provided it is at peace. However, there are also important differences between countries and these give real clues to the role of culture in affecting our happiness.

Why are some countries happier?

Countries vary hugely in their happiness levels, which shows there is no genetically determined set-point for the level of human happiness. If conditions improve, everyone in a country can become happier. The best source of data on country differences is the Gallup World Poll. These data have been the central source of information for the World Happiness Report, produced annually since 2012. The Report gives country rankings of happiness and trends in happiness for almost every country in the world. Not surprisingly, it attracts over 700,000 downloads a year. Table 2.1 below shows the latest rankings.

As in most other surveys, the happiest countries are those very egalitarian countries in Scandinavia. The Netherlands and Switzerland, two other vital democracies, are also in the top ten, together with three English-speaking countries: Australia, Canada and New Zealand. Then come a mixture of the main West European nations, including the UK, together with the United States. But interspersed among them are some Latin American countries, while lower down come other Latin American countries, together with Spain and Italy and some of the ex-Communist countries of Central Europe. Countries from the Gulf also figure quite high in the rankings. Moving to the bottom twenty, the great bulk of these countries are scenes of conflict – or have been in recent years.

So what, more generally, explains these rankings? John Helliwell has identified six factors which, when taken together, explain 76 per cent of the variance in average happiness across countries:[21]

- trust (the proportion of people who think 'most people can be trusted')
- generosity (the proportion who have donated money to a charity in the present month)
- social support (the proportion who have relatives or friends they can count on to help them whenever they need them)
- freedom (the proportion who are satisfied with their freedom to choose what they want to do with their life)
- health (years of healthy life expectancy)
- income (GDP per head).[22]

The effect of each variable is shown in Table 2.2 below. We can begin with trust. In some countries like Brazil almost no one trusts other people, while in Scandinavia it is around 70 per cent.[23] As Table 2.1 shows, a country where everyone trusts is 1 whole point happier (out of 10) than a country where no one trusts. Thus higher levels of trust help the Scandinavian countries to be happier. These are countries where the culture is more collaborative and less competitive than in the rest of Europe. Trust is also higher in Canada, Australia and New Zealand than in the UK and the USA.

Another key influence is social support – someone to rely on. This makes a huge difference. It tends to be high in Latin America, due to the close family ties that exist in that culture.[24] But freedom is also important,[25] as of course is health. And the absolute effect of income across countries is similar to its effect within countries.[26]

From this analysis we can see that social variables (as opposed to personal variables) also have an important effect on

1	Finland	7.8		Uzbekistan	6.2
	Denmark	7.6		Lithuania	6.1
	Norway	7.5		Colombia	6.1
	Iceland	7.5		Slovenia	6.1
	Netherlands	7.5		Nicaragua	6.1
	Switzerland	7.5		Kosovo	6.1
	Sweden	7.3		Argentina	6.1
	New Zealand	7.3		Romania	6.1
	Canada	7.3		Cyprus	6.0
10	Austria	7.2	50	Ecuador	6.0
	Australia	7.2		Kuwait	6.0
	Costa Rica	7.2		Thailand	6.0
	Israel	7.1		Latvia	5.9
	Luxembourg	7.1		South Korea	5.9
	United Kingdom	7.1		Estonia	5.9
	Germany	7.0		Jamaica	5.9
	Ireland	7.0		Mauritius	5.9
	Belgium	6.9		Japan	5.9
	United States	6.9		Honduras	5.9
20	Czech Republic	6.9	60	Kazakhstan	5.8
	United Arab Emirates	6.8		Bolivia	5.8
	Malta	6.7		Paraguay	5.8
	Mexico	6.6		Hungary	5.8
	France	6.6		North Cyprus	5.7
	Taiwan	6.4		Peru	5.7
	Chile	6.4		Portugal	5.7
	Guatemala	6.4		Russia	5.6
	Saudi Arabia	6.4		Philippines	5.6
	Qatar	6.4		Pakistan	5.6
30	Spain	6.4	70	Serbia	5.6
	Panama	6.3		Moldova	5.5
	Brazil	6.3		Libya	5.5
	Uruguay	6.3		Montenegro	5.5
	Singapore	6.3		Tajikistan	5.5
	El Salvador	6.3		Croatia	5.4
	Italy	6.2		Hong Kong	5.4
	Bahrain	6.2		Dominican Republic	5.4
	Slovakia	6.2		Bosnia & Herzegovina	5.4
	Trinidad and Tobago	6.2		Turkey	5.4
40	Poland	6.2	80	Malaysia	5.3

	Belarus	5.3			Kenya	4.5
	Greece	5.3			Mauritania	4.5
	Mongolia	5.3			Mozambique	4.5
	Macedonia	5.3			Tunisia	4.5
	Nigeria	5.3			Bangladesh	4.5
	Kyrgyzstan	5.3			Iraq	4.4
	Turkmenistan	5.2			Congo (Kinshasa)	4.4
	Algeria	5.2			Myanmar	4.4
	Morocco	5.2			Mali	4.4
90	Azerbaijan	5.2		130	Sierra Leone	4.4
	Morocco	5.2			Sri Lanka	4.4
	Lebanon	5.2			Chad	4.4
	Indonesia	5.2			Ukraine	4.3
	China	5.2			Ethiopia	4.3
	Vietnam	5.2			Swaziland	4.2
	Cameroon	5.0			Uganda	4.2
	Bulgaria	5.0			Egypt	4.2
	Ghana	5.0			Zambia	4.1
	Ivory Coast	4.9			Togo	4.1
100	Nepal	4.9		140	India	4.0
	Jordan	4.9			Liberia	4.0
	Benin	4.9			Comoros	4.0
	Congo (Brazzaville)	4.8			Madagascar	3.9
	Gabon	4.8			Lesotho	3.8
	Laos	4.7			Burundi	3.8
	South Africa	4.7			Zimbabwe	3.7
	Albania	4.7			Haiti	3.6
	Venezuela	4.7			Botswana	3.5
	Palestine	4.7			Syria	3.5
110	Senegal	4.7		150	Malawi	3.4
	Niger	4.7			Yemen	3.4
	Somalia	4.7			Rwanda	3.3
	Namibia	4.6			Tanzania	3.2
	Burkina Faso	4.6			Afghanistan	3.2
	Guinea	4.6			Central African Republic	3.1
	Armenia	4.6			South Sudan	2.9
	Iran	4.5				
	Guinea	4.5				
	Georgia	4.5				
120	Gambia	4.5				

Table 2.1 — Ranking of countries by their average happiness (on the scale 0–10)

Variable	Change in variable	Impact of change
Trust	100% v. 0%	0.98
Generosity	100% v. 0%	0.85
Social support	100% v. 0%	2.10
Freedom	100% v. 0%	1.27
Health	extra year	0.03
Income	doubles	0.25

Table 2.2
How is national happiness (0–10) affected by national variables?

our happiness. It really matters whether you can trust people, and have someone who will help you in times of trouble. This reminds us of the importance of those who set the tone for a society – the community leaders and the politicians.

But despite all this, some people maintain that each person has a set-point of happiness as a result of their genes. The huge international differences show just how false that belief is. Moreover, as we shall see in Chapter 11, when people move from one country to another, their happiness is often transformed. So we can indeed create a happier world.

Are we getting happier?

But are we actually getting happier? The answer is that it de-pends on where you live. In the US, people are no happier now than they were in the 1950s, despite huge improvements in living standards at least up to the 1970s.[27] In West Ger-many people are no happier than in the 1970s when records began.[28] And in China they are no happier than they were in 1990 when their records began.[29] However, in more countries than not, happiness rose from 1980 to 2007.[30] But since 2007 world happiness has stagnated: it has fallen in nearly as many countries as those where it has risen.[31]

What accounts for these facts? The first point to make about movements in happiness is that they are cyclical – happiness rises in economic booms and falls in recessions.[32] But does long-term economic growth increase happiness? This is still an unresolved issue. Richard Easterlin, using only countries with long time-series on happiness, claims that when you compare countries, there is no relation between their rate of economic growth and their increase in happiness.

If this is true, there are two obvious possible explanations. Either people are comparing themselves with other people whose incomes also rose, or they are simply adapting to higher income and taking it for granted. Our research group has examined both explanations and found more evidence of social comparison than of adaptation.[33]

However, two careful American researchers, Betsey Stevenson and Justin Wolfers, dispute Easterlin's original finding.[34] So the most we can say is that economic growth is no *guarantee* of increased happiness. We should surely welcome it, but only as one of a whole range of ways to make the world happier.

We should certainly not sacrifice too much else in the pursuit of higher income. And this is what seems to be happening. Worldwide there is an increase in stress. As Figure 2.3 shows, more and more people are saying 'Yes', when asked 'Did you experience a lot of stress yesterday?' Although the graph covers only the USA and Western Europe, the trend is worldwide, in an online annex.[35]

Conclusions

The science of happiness thus offers us the following new insights:

- Within countries, differences in happiness among adults are due to inner differences in mental and physical health as much as to the outer differences. And the most important outer differences are the quality of our human relationships at home, at work and in the community. Income inequality explains at most 2 per cent of the differences in happiness. Thus we need a new concept

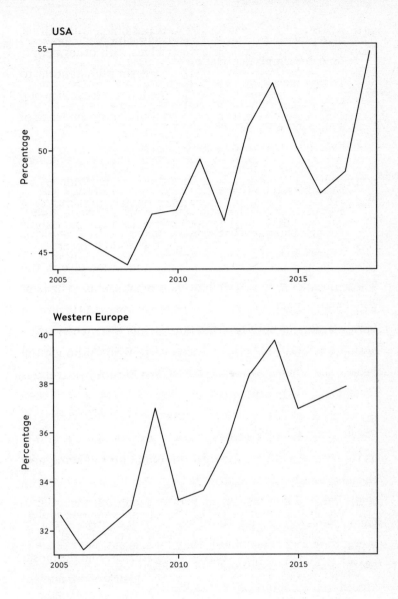

Figure 2.3
Stress is increasing (percentage saying 'I experienced a lot of stress yesterday')

of deprivation – it should mean deprivation of happiness (and not simply deprivation of income).

- To become a happy adult, it is more important to be a happy child than to get good grades. But schools have a huge influence on the happiness of their children.
- Everyone is affected by the overall institutions and ethos of their country. Countries are happier if (as in Scandinavia) there is a high level of trust, strong social support, personal freedom and low levels of corruption.
- Because happiness has so many causes, economic growth, though desirable, is no guarantee of rising happiness.

These insights throw fresh light on how we can improve our lives. They suggest major new areas where we need to develop better strategies both for individuals and for communities – action on child wellbeing, on wellbeing at work, on mental health, on families and on community cohesion.

But they do not tell us what exactly we should do in each of these areas. That is where experimental science comes in. This has made great strides in many areas of our social life, as we shall see in Part Two. But in none of these areas have the advances been more striking than in clinical psychology – the science of how we can gain control over our mental life. Closely related to that, there has been the growing rise in meditation and mindfulness, for which, again, there is a scientific basis. So techniques of mind-training are the third strand in the happiness revolution.

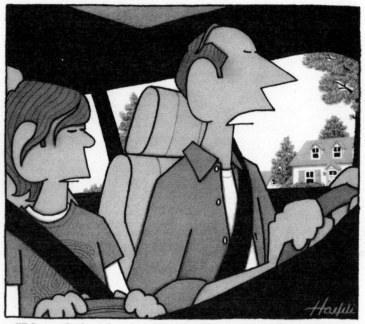

"If you bring joy and enthusiasm to everything you do, people will think you're crazy."

Training Our Thoughts and Our Feelings

Happy the Man, and happy he alone
He who can call today his own:
He, who secure within, can say,
Tomorrow do thy worst, for I have lived today.
— *from* Horace, Ode 29, translated by John Dryden[1]

In the 1960s Aaron Beck was a young psychiatrist who treated his depressed patients with Freudian psychoanalysis.[2] The idea was that depression was caused by repressed anger and could be treated by dream analysis in which the unconscious anger could be brought into consciousness and thus dispelled. Beck decided to test whether this was true, so he and his colleagues compared the dreams of depressed patients with those of other patients. And he found that they actually contained less anger than other people's dreams.

But they did contain many themes that were quite similar to those in their waking thoughts. The depressed patients had extremely pessimistic views of themselves, of the outside world, and of their own future. And those 'automatic negative thoughts' arose minute by minute in their waking life too. It was those thoughts that were maintaining the depression. Thus was born cognitive therapy – the idea that we can help people by helping them to observe and manage their thoughts. As Beck found, it was possible to empower the conscious mind enough to remove many depressions.

So that is what this chapter is about – the fact that we can train our minds by conscious processes, which, if all goes well, become so habitual that we hardly notice them. Psychological therapy works that way, so does 'positive psychology', and so does meditation. They are the next major element in the happiness revolution. To learn these skills some people need help from a therapist, but millions have taught themselves.

The new psychology

The first scientific breakthrough in psychology preceded cognitive therapy. In the 1960s a South African doctor called Joseph Wolpe found he could treat anxiety disorders by behavioural methods: he exposed people gradually to what they feared until the fear went away.[3] Gordon Paul then subjected these methods to the first systematic randomized experiment in clinical psychology.[4] In it people with a phobia about public speaking were treated either by systematic desensitization or by a Freudian insight-oriented therapy. The first of these therapies worked much better than the second.

Then in the 1970s Aaron Beck introduced cognitive therapy. Its basic idea is that thoughts affect feelings and vice versa, but the most effective way to break a negative cycle between thoughts and feelings is to address the thoughts. We can learn to observe our automatic negative thoughts, to challenge them and then to develop more positive thoughts.[5]

This idea has the widest possible relevance to all of us and how we can manage our emotional life.

Eventually the cognitive and behavioural strands came together, because much behavioural training also works through its effects on thoughts.[6] Thus was born **Cognitive Behavioural Therapy** (CBT). This is particularly effective in treating anxiety disorders, with 50–70 per cent recovery rates and very low relapse rates for those who recover. CBT is also effective in ending episodes of depression, with 50 per cent recovery rates during treatment and a halved rate of subsequent relapse. For depression, other effective psychological treatments also exist with good experimental evidence of success. For adults, these include interpersonal therapy, couples therapy and brief psychodynamic therapy, and specific forms of counselling are also recommended. For children with disturbed behaviour or ADHD, parent training has long-lasting effects, as has CBT for most other problems with children.

Unfortunately, however, few of these psychological therapies are widely available to most of those who need them. What is most widely available in the West – and is a major aspect of our new culture – is counselling of all types. This is an extremely positive development for at least two reasons. First, people are acknowledging their needs – the fact that we are all screwed up in some way or another. This is much better than pretending that we are all perfect. And, second, it implies that our mental processes are the central issue – how we think.

We can all improve our thoughts and thus our happiness. But this needs to be based on solid science. That is the message of *Emotional Intelligence*, popularized by Daniel Goleman in his book of 1995.[7] And it is the purpose of the new **Positive Psychology**, launched by Martin Seligman in 1998, as a means to greater happiness for everyone. Seligman had spent much of his life working on mental distress, but he now conjectured that the basic ideas of cognitive therapy could also be used to make all of us happier – whether we were initially distressed or not. So positive psychology starts with the idea that your thoughts affect your feelings. But it then focuses less on your negative thoughts and your personal weaknesses, and more on using your existing strengths in order to generate positive emotion. Seligman recommends a whole set of exercises for making yourself happier. These include two exercises around gratitude.[8] In one of them you write down each evening three things that went well during the day. And in another you write a letter of gratitude to someone whom you feel has really helped you in your life. Seligman and his academic colleagues have now trained a small army of positive psychologists, who are influencing individuals and policy-makers around the world.

These new developments are home-grown in the West. But equally profound in cultural terms has been the spread of ancient wisdom and practice from the East. The Western and Eastern strands have much in common, and they reinforce each other.[9]

The rise of meditation and mindfulness

In Hindu and Buddhist thought the central idea is the importance of the mind. It is your mental state that matters and you can learn to control it.

The first major wave of Eastern influence into the West

was in the swinging 60s, as part of the revolt of youth against conventional culture. The symbolic figure was the Hindu guru Maharishi Mahesh Yogi, who taught Transcendental Meditation (TM) as the route to a deeper level of consciousness – finding the beauty within. This practice involves sitting absolutely still and repeating a mantra. The Maharishi's many followers included the Beatles – this was the hippie generation.

But by the 1980s the economies of the US and Britain had become less buoyant – jobs were scarcer and neo-liberal philosophy was on the rise, led by President Ronald Reagan and Prime Minister Margaret Thatcher. The younger generation became more sober, but they too wanted good experiences. So the search for wellbeing ceased to be perceived as a drop-out, New Age activity and became instead a mainstream activity for people from all walks of life, from education to banking. Yoga became increasingly popular – for its physical benefits in the main, but also for its calming effect on the mind. And more and more people began to meditate.

Here the main influence in recent years has been Buddhism, with its clear philosophy of the working of the human mind. The leading figure is the Dalai Lama, the spiritual leader of the Tibetan people-in-exile and a deeply wise person with a great sense of fun. As he explains, everyone wants to be happy, but they are often deluded about what brings happiness. The greatest happiness comes not from getting, but from giving. And it also requires control of your own mental activity. This can be attained through the practice of meditation.

The most popular form of meditation in the West today

is probably mindfulness.[10] This means focusing your awareness on some aspect of the present moment, without judging it. For beginners the starting point is to focus on your
breathing. Attention then extends to the whole body, including any physical pain. From this it can move to your mental
activity – including any painful thoughts. Remarkably, when
these painful thoughts and sensations are just observed,
as if from the outside, they become less painful, less all-
consuming. The overall result from practising mindfulness
is greater peace of mind.

Unlike many other spiritual practices, mindfulness has
been subject to rigorous scientific evaluation, using randomized controlled trials that compare the happiness of participants with those of non-participants. These studies have
centred especially on the eight-session course known as
Mindfulness-Based Stress Reduction (MBSR), developed by
Jon Kabat-Zinn at the University of Massachusetts hospital
in Amherst.[11] Trials of MBSR have shown that four months
after the course, participants were less anxious compared
with those who had not taken part.[12] They also had better
brain measurements and a much stronger immunity to flu
(after a flu jab). Other trials have shown that mindfulness
also protects against depression.[13] MBSR courses have now
been taken by over a million people and many more have
learned their mindfulness in other ways, including via some
wonderful apps like Headspace. Most practitioners will say
that mindfulness is more than just a form of meditation –
it's a way of life, a way of noticing and appreciating the
world around you and inside you.

The appeal of mindfulness is partly because of its

non-religious, semi-medical character: it overlaps significantly with cognitive therapy and positive psychology. But, according to critics, both mindfulness and positive psychology (if narrowly conceived) lack one key element: altruism.[14] They are mainly about how to make yourself happier, not other people. By contrast, altruism is about caring for others.

Altruism

Matthieu Ricard is an expert in altruism and a Buddhist monk in the Tibetan tradition. He practises Compassion Meditation. When you meet him, he is wearing his robes and you would not believe he was once a promising French molecular biologist. At the age of twenty-six he moved to the Himalayas to be near his spiritual teacher. He hardly visited the West again for the next twenty-five years until he became a part-time French interpreter for the Dalai Lama.

From his early childhood, the Dalai Lama had a strong interest in Western science. As a boy (and at the same time Head of State) he insisted on dismantling his official car to find out how it worked – and then reassembling it. But he was, and remains, a deeply contemplative person, meditating for five hours each day. So he naturally came to wonder if Western science confirms the Buddhist theory of the mind.

To investigate this, the Dalai Lama has been meeting regularly for thirty years with Western scientists, including Richard Davidson of the University of Wisconsin, to discuss the similarities between Buddhist philosophy and Western cognitive psychology and neuroscience.[15] As a result of this contact with the Dalai Lama, Davidson has been leading a research programme into the neuroscience of meditation.

At one point in this research, Matthieu Ricard was wired up and, as a result of his exceptional brain measurement, he has been called 'the happiest man in the world'.

The meetings with the Dalai Lama, run by the Mind & Life Institute, have resulted in a number of excellent publications on such issues as the control of destructive emotions and the practice of caring.[16] A key theme of all these books is the necessity for altruism. Neuroscientists have now confirmed that altruism is an intrinsic element in human nature and have found that the human brain includes at least three important circuits. The first two are well recognized in neo-conservative philosophy: they are the 'appetitive' and 'aversive' circuits. But there is also a third circuit which is 'affiliative', or, to use plain English, loving.[17]

Like all our faculties, this 'affiliative' circuit only exists as a potential attribute – it has to be actively cultivated. So our aim should be to carve into ourselves the disposition to love those who come our way. In Ricard's words, the aim must be 'unconditional benevolence'.

Conclusions: the new culture

Thus the new culture that is emerging includes a revolutionary insight – that we can gain control over our mental life, at least to some extent. We are not simply receptacles for our emotions; we can make ourselves mentally fit. We can work out mentally, just as we can work out physically.

Physical fitness took off first, but mental health is following hard on its heels. This concept of mind-training offers new hope to those who are struggling with their mental health and is central to treatments such as CBT. But it also offers liberation to all of us. The gentler culture includes at least three complementary elements:

- The new psychology, which combines modern science and ancient wisdom to help us care for ourselves
- Mindfulness, which provides a regular practice that gives us control over our mental life
- Compassion, which makes us care for others and, through that, for ourselves.

This is not a philosophy of selfish hedonism, but neither is it an austere philosophy of self-sacrifice. We need to care for ourselves, to have fun *and* to care for others. A wonderful teacher whose work includes all three elements is the Zen Buddhist monk Thich Nhat Hanh. Born in Vietnam, he tried unsuccessfully to mediate in the Vietnam War, and since then he has lived in exile in France. In 1975 he published *The Miracle of Mindfulness* – which includes the clearest possible account of the link between mindfulness (as a practice) and ethical living.[18]

He states, 'With mindfulness, concentration, and insight, you are capable of generating a feeling of joy and happiness whenever you want. With the energy of mindfulness, you can also handle a painful feeling or emotion.'[19] You can, he says, embrace your suffering. According to Thich Nhat Hanh, people say, 'Don't just sit there, do something.' On the contrary, he says, 'Don't just do something, sit there.' Learn to be, as well as to do. The present is all we have. Learn to be present in the present moment. 'Time is not money; time is life.'

*

Let me end with the Dalai Lama. Picture him waking each morning at 3.30 a.m. – wherever he is – and beginning to meditate. Each day he begins with the following prayer:[20]

> May I be a guard for those who need protection
> A guide for those on the path
> May I be a lamp in the darkness
> A resting place for the weary
> A healing medicine for all who are sick
> A vase of plenty, a tree of miracles
> And for the boundless multitudes of living beings
> May I bring sustenance and awakening.

So now we have the basis for a more spiritual culture – one where people deliberately cultivate in themselves a calm, joyful and loving frame of mind. This includes proper care of our inner selves and a strong desire to help others – to make a difference. Two key features are calm and caring.

Calm: We cultivate the means to calm ourselves and to accept our discontents. We appreciate the wonders of life and savour each moment.

Caring: We deeply desire the happiness of others and aim to promote it (unconditional benevolence). We truly believe that our own feelings are no more important than anyone else's, and we try to feel what others feel.[21]

This is not about opting out. It is a philosophy of realistic engagement. As the Serenity Prayer says, we need the courage to change the bad things we can change, the serenity to accept the bad things we cannot change, and the wisdom to know the difference.

But what are the prospects for this new, more generous culture – this New Enlightenment? Are the cross-winds too strong? As we shall see in the next chapter, cross-winds abound. But there are also strong currents in our favour.

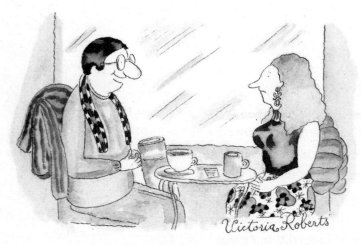

"I've tried a lot of life strategies, and being completely
self-serving works best for me."

Can the Happiness Movement Succeed?

> One of the things I can't stand about this town is the back-stabbing. Where I grew up, we're front-stabbers.
> — Anthony Scaramucci, 2017

There are two opposing strands in human nature. One says, 'I am at the centre of the universe and my needs come first.' The other says, 'I owe so much to others and I must give back.' One stresses the differences between my own needs and wants and those of others. The other stresses the similarities and what we all have in common. The relative strengths of these two influences is determined to a large extent by the prevailing culture in which we live.

The rise of excessive individualism

In modern culture the selfish strand is now legitimized as never before. The chief goal on offer to young people is success relative to others – better grades, higher pay, more friends and greater fame. This is especially so in the United States. For example, among college entrants more and more of them think it is important to be very well off financially and fewer think it essential to develop a philosophy of life (see Figure 4.1). Increasingly, young people compete in every possible avenue of life.

These trends in youth culture have been studied intensively by Jean Twenge at San Diego State University.[1] She finds that 31 per cent of high school students expect to be famous one day,[2] and an increasing percentage of college entrants think they are above average.[3] Similar narcissistic tendencies are exemplified in the candidate whom American electors knowingly chose as President in 2016. As Donald Trump elegantly put it, 'Show me someone without an ego and I'll show you a loser.' Or, as the director of counselling at the University of Nebraska put it, 'If you don't have a me-first attitude, you won't succeed.'[4]

Such attitudes are not much fun for other people. They are also bad advice. For research shows that successful businessmen are no more narcissistic or self-confident than average – they are good builders of teams.[5]

However, it is easy to see how the Me-First philosophy can take root, unless constantly challenged by a more unselfish view of the purpose of life. After all we mostly live in large cities in which no one has any automatic position. To do anything worthwhile you have to establish your position, and this requires an element of self-promotion. But what matters is the purpose behind it. If your purpose is to be useful and create happiness, that's fine. But if it is to come out on top, that's not good – ruthless competition is one of the most powerful destroyers of happiness.

Me-First individualism has grown fastest in the USA, but it has increased everywhere. Scandinavian countries have been famous for teaching the pro-social values of respect and

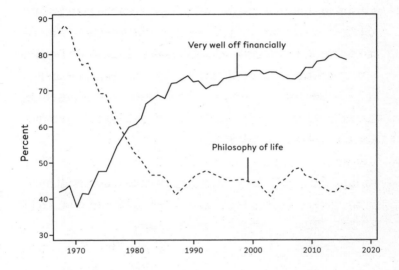

Figure 4.1
US students have become more materialistic (percentage saying each goal is essential or very important)

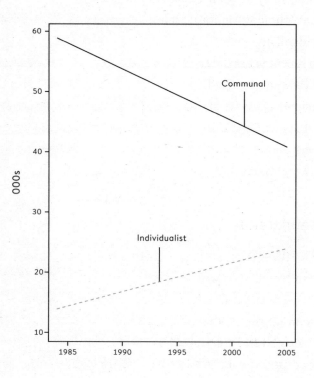

Figure 4.2
A Norwegian newspaper reflects increasing individualism and
reduced communal values (numbers of words of each type per year)

fellow-feeling to their citizens, but even in Norway there is evidence of change. One study by their main national newspaper counted the frequency of communal words (such as 'shared', 'duty', 'equality') and of individualistic words (such as 'me', 'choice', 'rights'). Figure 4.2 tells the tale of growing individualism.

In recent years the rise in competitiveness has been made much worse by the advent of social media. We discuss this in Chapter 13. As we show, social media has encouraged self-advertisement and made more young people feel inadequate, anxious, depressed and 'left out'. In addition it has encouraged populism, which is an increasing challenge to a cohesive and loving society.

Hopeful trends

None of these trends will be easy to alter. But there are many hopeful trends too, both among citizens and among policy-makers. We have already documented many of them. Let me mention three other encouraging trends. The first is the spectacular **fall in crime** of all kinds in recent decades in most advanced countries.[6] This new degree of gentleness is one of the least noticed and least well-understood changes of our time, but it is deeply significant.

My own guess is that it reflects the **increased influence of women in our society**: women commit fewer crimes than men do, and they tend to avoid men who are criminals.[7] Moreover, most women care more about inner feelings than men do on average, while typically men have been more focused on externals.[8] This shift of perspective is central to the happiness movement which is about the overarching importance of our feelings – our quality of life as we actually experience it.

A third trend is partly helpful and partly not so. It is the growing **toleration of diversity**. That has already trans-formed the happiness of minority groups, including people who are LGBT, disabled or (until recently) immigrant.[9] But it can also involve another not so good attitude – lack of con-cern. In other words, 'You do your thing and I'll do mine. I won't bother you, but I won't engage with you either.' When I first came to London in the 1950s, people talked to each other on the buses. Now, when you sit next to someone, they look away.[10] That is not so good. We want a society which is toler-ant, but also friendly and compassionate. Making this change will play an important part in producing a happier society.

So the ground is fertile. Contrary to popular belief, sat-isfaction with life is not low by historical standards in the West, except in the USA, Italy and Greece (see Chapter 12). Populism is a venting of dissatisfaction which has been there for a long time, but has not been previously expressed. It is being expressed now because of the discredited credentials of the elites from 2008 onwards and the legitimation of rude-ness by social media.

But the dissatisfaction is real and requires urgent reforms of social and economic policy. These should of course be based on the Happiness Principle. But are our leaders up for implementing the Happiness Principle?

Are governments listening?

Our first hero in the political sphere is Enrico Giovannini, an enterprising Italian who was once the Chief Statistician of the OECD. The OECD is the club of rich nations, and it was the OECD that started the standard measurement of GDP in the 1950s. But in 2004 Giovannini persuaded the OECD to open a public debate on the nature of progress – the issue often referred to as 'Beyond GDP'. Since then the OECD has held another five major conferences to 'push forward the boundaries of wellbeing measurement and policy'. In 2012 it recommended that its member countries should measure the subjective wellbeing of their adult population each year, and most of them now do so.[11] In 2015 measurement of life-satisfaction was extended to fifteen-year-olds in the OECD survey known as PISA (Programme for International Student Assessment). In 2016, remarkably, the OECD first said that we should 'put people's wellbeing at the centre of govern-ments' efforts'.[12] And in 2019 it held a special meeting of governments to consider how far each government plans to use wellbeing as the goal of its policies.[13]

The UN too has been active. In 2012 it established an annual International Day of Happiness (20 March), and the UN General Assembly called upon its members to give more attention to the happiness of their people.[14] At the same time a leading development economist Jeffrey Sachs, who was an adviser to the UN Secretary General, proposed the idea of an annual World Happiness Report. This is now presented each year at the UN. In addition, the annual World Government Summit in Dubai now hosts the presentation of a more policy-oriented Global Happiness and Wellbeing Policy Report. But what are individual governments actually doing about all this?

In January 2019, Jacinda Ardern, the Prime Minister of New Zealand, was addressing world leaders at Davos. She announced that her government had adopted wellbeing as its goal and would use it as the basis of her forthcoming budget for wellbeing. So New Zealand became the first Western country to formally target wellbeing.[15] In the meantime many other countries, local governments and cities have been taking steps in the same direction, including the governments of France and Britain.[16] In 2008 the French President, Nicolas Sarkozy, set up a distinguished commission to report on the measurement of progress,[17] and, following on from that, French law (like that of Sweden) now requires all major policy changes to be analysed for their impact on (among other things) wellbeing.

Britain has in many ways gone further than this. It was the first country to measure national subjective wellbeing as an official statistic, and its top civil servant for many years, Gus O'Donnell, pushed for subjective wellbeing as a goal of government policy. After leaving government he chaired a committee that produced the best available account of how that might be done.[18] So in Britain many central government departments and many local governments now include 'wellbeing' divisions. And the 'Green Book',[19] which describes how policy proposals should be appraised, has 'social wellbeing' as its objective and recommends the use of data on subjective wellbeing wherever willingness-to-pay cannot be used as a measure of benefit.

At the more local level, many governments of regions and cities in different countries have gone just about as far as New Zealand has. They include Jalisco (in Mexico), Andhra Pradesh (in India), Scotland, and the city of Bristol (in the UK).[20]

The movement for change is strong. Governments make the decisions, but they are of course responding to a growing alteration in the public mood. This change is also reflected in the increasing number of citizens' events directed at the goal of happiness, above all the annual World Happiness Summit held in Miami.

Conclusions

So will the happiness revolution succeed? I believe it will.

- On the one side there is still a strong tide of excessive individualism. And this is now augmented by social media, which encourages yet more self-promotion.
- But on the other side there is an increasing gentleness in society – less crime, greater gender equality, and a greater toleration of diversity.
- Moreover, governments are listening. A few countries and regional governments have adopted happiness as their overarching goal. But, in many more, happiness is increasingly used as a key measure of success.

In struggles over culture, change can come quite quickly. The last forty years have seen extraordinary changes in public attitudes to gender equality; sex outside marriage; cigarette smoking; gay and lesbian relationships; and, most recently, issues such as sexual harassment, child abuse and domestic violence.[21] Similarly, in the forty years after the French Revolution there were astonishingly rapid changes in attitudes to slavery, gambling, drinking, extra-marital sex, and duelling.[22] So there is no reason why, in less than forty years from now, the culture of gentleness could not displace the dominant culture of excessive individualism. But how can each one of us help to make this happen?

PART TWO

Who Can Do What?

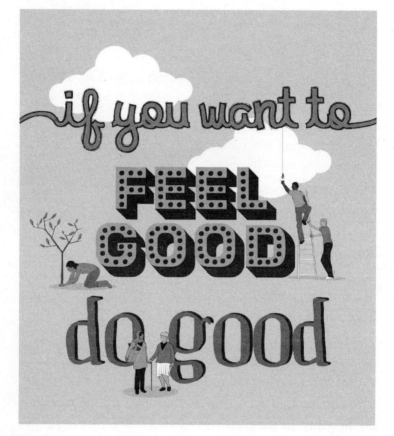

Each of Us

Without ethical culture there is no salvation for humanity.
— Albert Einstein[1]

In 2015 the Dalai Lama was in London launching a new course called 'Exploring What Matters'. At one point a middle-aged woman came on to the stage. She was in pain and on crutches. For years she had been mostly bedridden and often depressed. But then she happened to hear about the course and enrolled locally. It changed her life. She realized that, by helping others like herself, she could give meaning to her life. The Dalai Lama embraced her. Later on, he was asked, 'What is the most important thing for a happy life?' Without hesitation, he replied, 'Warm heart'.

In the end it is each of us as individuals who will determine the levels of happiness in our society – by everything we do. It is not easy to live well, but it is very much easier if you are in regular contact with people who are trying to do the same. In the West this used to happen when people went to church. They were reminded that they were not the centre of the universe: there was something bigger than them. And they were inspired, uplifted and comforted. They re-established contact with their 'better selves'.

The moral vacuum

But today very few Europeans go to church, and even in the USA religion has been losing its hold (see Figure 5.1).[2] This is one of the most profound changes of our age. People no longer define ethical behaviour as conforming to the will of God. To some extent the old rules of behaviour – based on religion – persist, but their hold is weakening. Back in 1952 one half of all Americans thought people led 'as good lives – moral and honest – as they used to'. There was no majority for the view that 'things are going to the dogs'. But by 1998 there was a three-to-one majority for precisely that view – that people are less moral than they used to be.

Clearly there has developed, to a degree, a moral vacuum into which have stepped some dreadful ideas. Many of these ideas are highly individualistic, with an excessive emphasis on competition and on personal success as the key goal in life. In that view each person's main obligation is to themselves. An extreme proponent of this view is the writer Ayn Rand, who became the favourite guru of Alan Greenspan and later of Donald Trump.[3] In her world individuals do of course collaborate on occasion, but only when it is in their own individual interest to do so. There is no concept of the common good, and life is largely a struggle for places on the ladder of success. But such a struggle is a zero-sum game, since if one person rises, another must fall. In such a world it is impossible for everyone to become happier. For that to happen, it has to be through a positive-sum game where success for one brings success for others.

So we need a new ethics that incorporates the best values

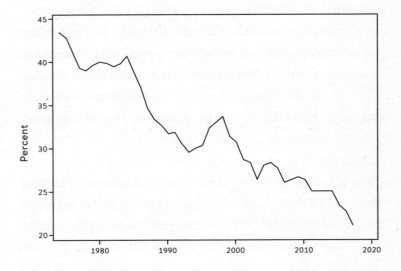

Figure 5.1
Percentage saying that they had a great deal of confidence in the church or organized religion (USA)

to be found in all religions, but which is equally convincing to people with no religious faith at all. As the Dalai Lama has put it, 'For all its benefits in offering moral guidance and meaning in life, religion is no longer adequate as a basis for ethics. Many people no longer follow any religion. In addition, in today's secular and multicultural societies, any religion-based answer to the problem of our neglect of inner values could not be universal, and so would be inadequate. We need an approach to ethics that can be equally acceptable to those with religious faith and those without. We need a secular ethics.'[4]

What should it be based on? It has to be based on our Ethical Principle – that each of us should try to create the most happiness we can in the world, especially among those who are least happy. This principle has a universal appeal, to people of faith as well as those of no faith. In the language of Christians, Jews and Muslims, it embodies the commandment to love your neighbour as yourself. In the language of Buddhists, Confucians and Hindus, it encompasses the principle of compassion – that in all our dealings we should truly wish for the happiness of all of those we can affect, and that we should cultivate in ourselves an attitude of unconditional benevolence.[5]

This faith allows us to think of ourselves as well as others. But, since there are so many more others, it strongly encourages us to achieve our own happiness in large part by contributing to the happiness of others.

No belief system can flourish without institutions that embody it – gatherings where people can meet regularly to reinforce their commitment to live well. But there are as yet surprisingly few secular institutions which attempt to fill the void left by the retreat of religion. When I was a student at

Cambridge, I was a founder member of the Cambridge Humanists and I hoped that Humanist associations worldwide would inspire people to lead good lives. But mostly they have concentrated instead on the less inspiring role of criticizing religion.

In the West the most obvious non-theistic groups that meet regularly around the central issues of life are Buddhists and mindfulness groups.[6] There are also huge numbers of charitable organizations. Some have specific benevolent purposes (like Alcoholics Anonymous, the Red Cross and countless forms of volunteering). Others have wider purposes but a restricted membership. But there are very few secular organizations which can be compared with the churches, whose purpose is the whole of life and whose membership is open to all.

That is why in 2011 we founded **Action for Happiness**, a secular movement for a happier society. The patron is the Dalai Lama, and members make the following pledge: 'I will try to create more happiness and less unhappiness in the world around me.' So far, over 150,000 people from 175 countries have made that pledge – in other words they will live according to our Ethical Principle. And over a million other people are following the Action for Happiness message on Facebook, which shows the hunger that exists for these ideas.

But how in practice does Action for Happiness help people to live better and more fulfilling lives?

- First, it offers them Ten Keys to Happier Living (online and in book form).[7]
- Second, it offers an eight-session course on Exploring What Matters, where people can reflect on how our Ethical Principle can be applied in their lives.

- Third, it is forming thousands of groups worldwide who meet regularly to inspire each other, using standard materials which the movement provides.

Ten Keys to Happier Living

The Ten Keys are a guide to behaviour and attitudes conducive to a happy society, based on the evidence of modern psychology.[8] But they also embody much of the ancient wisdom found in Buddhism, Christianity, Confucianism, Graeco-Roman philosophy, Hinduism, Islam and Judaism. In all of these traditions there is a common core of teaching about how human beings should manage their mental lives, and that is what the Ten Keys are ultimately about – the management of our mental lives.[9]

All ten keys are shown in Figure 5.2, and the first letters of each key spell 'GREAT DREAM'. Those in the top section (GREAT) were first constructed in response to a question from the British government: 'If five fruit and vegetables a day are good for your physical health, what five things each day are good for your mental health?'[10] So the Daily Five are behaviours which should be undertaken at least once a day. But equally important are our 'habits of mind' – our basic philosophy of life. These comprise the bottom half of the figure and spell the word 'DREAM'.

It is natural to ask how these different elements relate to each other: which, if any, has priority? I will give my own answer to that question. Underlying all of the keys is a positive frame of mind – a habit of looking for the best in a situation, and the best in another person. Without this, nothing goes well. For example, the psychologist John Gottman has

GIVING	Do things for others
RELATING	Connect with people
EXERCISING	Take care of your body
AWARENESS	Live life mindfully
TRYING OUT	Keep learning new things
DIRECTION	Have goals to look forward to
RESILIENCE	Find ways to bounce back
EMOTIONS	Look for what's good
ACCEPTANCE	Be comfortable with who you are
MEANING	Be part of something bigger

Figure 5.2
Ten Keys to Happier Living

shown that in happy marriages people make at least five positive comments to each other for every negative one, while in failing marriages the ratio is less than one to one.[11]

Human nature includes both positive and negative strands. In early human life in the savannah the negative strand was crucial. You always had to look out for threats and dangers in the world around. If you did not, you got eaten and failed to reproduce. Today, we have far fewer threats to our survival; but we still interpret as threats things which are not. In the English language, 62 per cent of the emotions for which words exist are negative emotions.[12] Negativity affects our willingness to reach out to other people and to new experiences. And it affects our response to genuine adversity. So if we want to be happy we have to consciously strengthen the positive side of ourselves. There is an old Cherokee story: an old man tells his grandson, 'There is a fight inside you between two wolves – one is selfish and the other is loving.' 'But,' says the boy, 'which wolf will win?' To which the old man replies, 'The one you feed.'[13]

Thus a positive approach is what can help us with each of the keys. Starting with our 'habits of mind', positive thought obviously generates positive emotion. Gratitude exercises are strongly recommended along the lines proposed by Martin Seligman (and many ancient sages before him).[14] A positive frame of mind also generates the right responses to adversity. Resilience comes from treating a setback as a challenge, and trying to accept it as such. Positive thinking also means that we accept ourselves and we accept others. We avoid constant comparisons between us and them, and we learn to forgive. Acceptance does not mean passivity – it provides the firm foundation for action. For this we need an inspiring purpose, a direction and meaning in our lives.[15] So our general habit of mind should be one of compassion – both to others and to ourselves.[16]

This in turn affects our daily actions. So, turning to the Daily Five, the first place goes to giving. This is for two reasons: it helps the helped, and it helps the giver. As Portia put it in *The Merchant of Venice* when she described mercy, 'It is twice blessed; It blesseth him that gives and him that takes.' Next comes relating. We are deeply social animals and we are desperate to be loved and appreciated. The best way to be loved and appreciated by someone is to care for them – to help them, and make them feel better each time they see you. At the centre of any successful relationship is the heartfelt desire for the other's wellbeing. Help that is given for the sake of a good turn in response (reciprocity) is less satisfying than help given out of the goodness of your heart (altruism). What is required in our relations with others is more than respect or toleration; it is heart-felt goodwill.

Through practice, we can increase the level of our goodwill. The leading expert on positivity, Barbara Fredrickson of the University of North Carolina, has studied the effects of Loving Kindness Meditation, otherwise known as Compassion Meditation or Mettā. In this meditation the participants cultivate good feelings in succession, first for themselves, and then for a loved one, then for an enemy and then for humankind. The results are increased positive emotion, increased flows of the feel-good hormone, oxytocin, and improved tone in the vagus nerve which controls the heart rate.[17]

Positivity also makes it easier to practise mindful

awareness. Meditation may help some people, but many of the most mindful people have never meditated. It is a matter of living more in the present and appreciating every good aspect of your surroundings and your life. Finally, we need the habit of exploration (trying out) – both mental curiosity and physical discovery – and the habit of physical exercise, on which so much has already been written.[18]

There are of course serious people who question the whole concept of positive thinking. For example, in her book *Smile or Die*, Barbara Ehrenreich prefers 'realistic thinking'.[19] But there doesn't need to be a conflict between being positive and being realistic. If we are to help other people, we need to be totally realistic about their situation. But when it comes to ourselves, we can choose what to focus on. If the external situation is really bad, we should try to change it. But if our life is the usual mixture of good and bad, it will be better for us (and for those around us) if we focus mainly on the good. Let's celebrate the glass half-full.

Action for Happiness groups

How can people be helped to practise the wisdom of the Ten Keys? The wisdom is on the Action of Happiness website and in Vanessa King's fine book on the Ten Keys. It is also reflected in the daily online calendars which are based on one Key per month and provide a helpful thought for each day.[20]

But almost anything really important is best done face to face with other people. That is the point of the course known as Exploring What Matters and of the Action for Happiness groups that emerge from it. Exploring What Matters is an eight-session course of two hours each week that surveys the great issues of living: what we are aiming at; what makes us happy; how we can calm our minds; how we can make others happy; how we can have good relationships at home and at work. Each course is led by two volunteers who are screened and supported from the centre. For each session a set of materials is provided and there is a standard format: a mindfulness period, followed by a video talk by an expert; then a review of scientific evidence; followed by a discussion of how this fits your experience and what action you will take as a result.

The Exploring What Matters course was launched by the Dalai Lama in London's Lyceum Theatre in 2015. It has proved remarkably successful. By mid-2019 over 300 courses had been held in sixteen countries with 5,000 participants. In addition there has been a scientific evaluation of the effects of the course. This trial involved 146 participants, half of whom were randomly chosen to be controls on a wait-list. The results were remarkable.[21] Two months after the course, people who took it were nearly a whole point higher in life-satisfaction (0–10) than if they had not taken the course. This is larger than the effect when an unemployed person gets a job – it is a big effect.

Another way of seeing the size of this effect is to ask if a person with average happiness took this course, where would she end up in the ranking of happiness? The answer is that she would probably rise from 50th place (with 100 being the highest rank) to 74th place – she would rise by 24 'percentage points'. This is often a very useful way of reporting the impact of a change and we shall use it frequently in this book.[22] It is used in Figure 5.3 below, which also shows

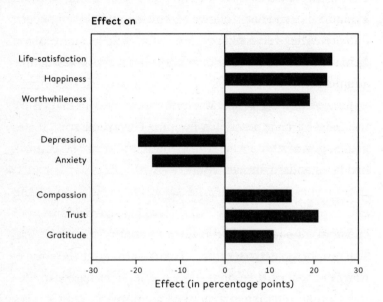

Effect on

Figure 5.3
The Exploring What Matters course has big effects
(two months later)

the dramatic effects of Exploring What Matters courses on mental health and on pro-social attitudes.

The success of the course is due not only to its powerful content, but also to two other features. There is no fee for the course – people give what they can afford or choose to give – so it attracts a huge cross-section of people, both rich and poor (as do churches), and disproportionately large numbers of people who are either very unhappy or very happy. Secondly, all of them are there on the basis of complete equality, including the volunteer leaders of the course. When asked about the impact of the course on their lives, an average of 97 per cent said it was positive. And, once people have completed the course, they are encouraged to create a local group which meets regularly following a standard format.

Related secular movements

There are of course other secular movements which share many of the objectives of the Action for Happiness groups. Many of them only teach courses rather than meeting regularly on an ongoing basis.[23] But some, like Buddhist and mindfulness groups, also meet regularly.

One movement with objectives similar to Action for Happiness is **Sunday Assembly**. Founded in 2013, these groups meet weekly, often with hundreds of participants. Their motto is 'Live better; help often; wonder more' and the theme of their meetings is celebration. Each meeting lasts roughly an hour, with a standard format including talks, singing and readings. The meetings are led by local leaders who have received an eight-session training webinar. Currently there are seventy Sunday Assemblies around the world.

Another recent movement has a particularly impressive record of growth: the **Art of Living Foundation**. This movement for harmonious and ethical living was founded in 1981 by Sri Sri Ravi Shankar, a wise Indian guru with a wonderful twinkle in his eyes.[24] The centrepiece of his teaching is the Happiness Course, which teaches a strenuous form of breathing. He also has his own version of meditation which is a modified version of TM, where the mind rests rather than concentrates. These two practices are the central features of group meetings of the Art of Living Foundation. The movement now has 10,000 groups worldwide. Unlike Action for Happiness, it is led by trained teachers, while Action for Happiness prefers volunteers, because this establishes an amazing atmosphere of equality and sharing during a meeting, which can be very uplifting.

The oldest movement of all is the **humanist movement** or the closely related ethical societies that exist worldwide.[25] They are of course the source of many of the ideas in this book, and they offer many excellent events such as lectures and humanist weddings and funerals. But they have not really satisfied the needs of millions of people to meet regularly in order to be strengthened, supported, comforted and uplifted. We need new organizations to do this.

Effective Altruism

There is one other issue for us as individuals: what should we do with our money? If we are relatively well-off, we could almost certainly do more good by giving some of our money away – that is, more good to others than the cost to us and our families.

One obvious target is poorer people in Third World

countries.[26] But what form should the aid take? There is a movement called **Effective Altruism**, which encourages people to make choices in life so as to maximize happiness all round.[27] So when giving money to charity, they advise giving to organizations that produce the biggest increase in happiness-years for every dollar they receive. To facilitate this, the website of Give Well, based in San Francisco, shows how different charities compare in terms of cost-effectiveness.[28] It shows, for example, that malaria and de-worming charities give excellent value for money. Another organization called **80,000 Hours** urges people to choose their careers so as to create the most happiness for present and future generations.[29] As that organization points out, for some people the most effective choice is to make a lot of money and then give most of it away.

Conclusions

A new culture has to be based on individuals – what we each value and how we behave.

- We need to address the moral vacuum which has been left by the retreat of religion. Where egotism has replaced it, we need instead the generous philosophy embodied in the Happiness Principle.
- To live well, we need to cultivate the positive side of our nature which can nourish us and help us reach out to others.
- For many people it will help to belong to a community of people, like Action for Happiness, who share our outlook.

Together we can build a happier society. But each of us will contribute in our own unique way. So what can people in different occupations do to make the world a happier place?

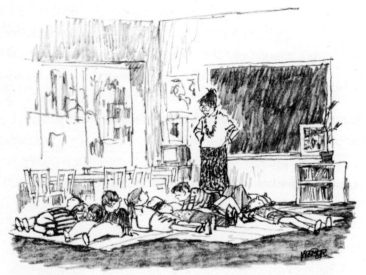

"The first one to fall asleep gets today's competitive-edge award."

Teachers

If you think you've got a problem, you should see the head.
— Notice in school staff room

Schools matter

Sceptics question whether teachers can make children happy. But the evidence shows that they can. The children born in 1991–2 in Bristol, England, have been followed up each year to see how they are faring. The researchers measured their happiness at age sixteen and, to explain it, they collected information about the children's parents, as well as about the primary and secondary schools they attended.

What they discovered was remarkable. How happy children are at sixteen depends as much on which secondary school they are at as on everything we know about their parents.[1] It is also profoundly affected by which primary school they attended all those years earlier. The findings are shown in Figure 6.1 below. This gives partial correlation coefficients which, as we explained earlier, reflect how far each factor contributes independently to the overall variation in happiness at age sixteen. The top row shows the effect of a weighted average of the measured characteristics of the parents. The

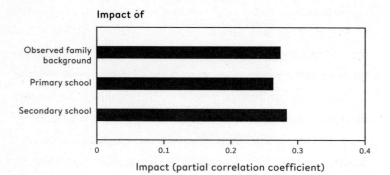

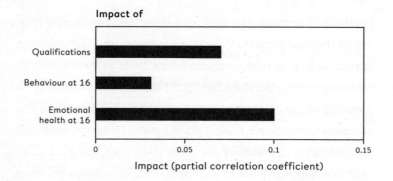

Figure 6.1
(*top*) What predicts happiness at age sixteen?
(*bottom*) What in childhood predicts a happy adult?

next row shows the influence of the primary school the student went to, and the bottom row shows the influence of the secondary school they attended.[2]

So schools make a huge difference to children's happiness at sixteen. They also have a significant impact on their behaviour. In fact they make about as much difference to their happiness and their behaviour as to their academic performance.

And so do individual teachers. In primary schools children are taught mainly by one teacher over the whole school year, so that in the Bristol survey we can trace how each teacher affected the happiness of the children in their care over the year. We found that the teacher made a greater difference to the children's happiness than to their performance in maths.[3] Remarkably, we can also see the long-lasting effect of individual primary school teachers on the children they taught, right up to the age of twenty.[4]

But how well, one might ask, does a child's happiness predict her subsequent happiness as an adult? Or shouldn't schools concentrate mainly on 'what they do best' – academic learning? The answer is a clear 'No'. For the best predictor of a happy adult life is a happy childhood. This emerges clearly from Figure 6.1. Here we have stacked the cards strongly in favour of academic qualifications, by including all qualifications up to the PhD. But all these qualifications contribute less to a happy life than one measure of emotional health taken at the age of sixteen.

Thus schools are crucial to a happy society, as of course are parents (see Chapter 9). But schools may be easier to influence, which is why we discuss them first.

Are things moving in the right direction?

So how well are schools doing at this job? Since parents want their children to be happy, you might think that happiness would be an explicit goal of every school.[5] In some it is, but in many it is not. And, if anything, the trend is in the wrong direction – with schools becoming ever more like exam factories. The situation differs between countries, but in England each year the exam results lead to published league tables of schools, ranked according to their academic performance. These scores become the outcome by which teachers are judged. The result is that the teachers get stressed, and from them (and from some parents) the pressure passes to the children. Children are often taught simply what they need to know for the test. This is hardly the way to train inquisitive minds that will go on learning joyfully throughout life. It is not even the best way to help children through exams.

For all the evidence shows that **happy children learn better**. This evidence is not simply correlational – it emerges from hundreds of interventions designed to make children happier, and which also make them do better at their academic work.[6]

In many countries test mania is affecting children of all ages. It underlies some aspects of the movement in support of 'early intervention'. The main impulse here is a well-placed worry about the academic development of children from poor families.[7] But the solution offered may not be the best one. Typically, the aim is to make children school-ready by the age of five so that they can learn to read as early as possible. But there is little evidence that being pushed to read earlier makes children better readers at the age of, say, eleven.[8] Indeed, many of the countries with the best reading results at age eleven start reading at six or seven, when many children find learning easier.[9] Starting earlier can just make them more anxious about reading.

At the same time, play has become devalued. Recently, England's Chief Inspector of Schools wrote to pre-school teachers saying that play should be 'teacher-led'. On the contrary, it is vital for children to organize their own play. This is confirmed in an interesting experiment on rats. Some of the young rats were reared with other equally rambunctious young rats; they experienced many a tumble. Other rats in the experiment were reared with rats made docile with drugs. When they became adults, the young rats who had experienced the rougher play were less anxious and more exploratory than those who had been protected from tumbles.[10]

Moving on to older children, there is a sorry tale from the influential PISA study of young people aged fifteen, conducted by the OECD.[11] In the last survey, over a third of all the young people in OECD countries said, 'I get very tense when I study'. As Table 6.1 shows, OECD students feel much less comfortable at school now than they did ten years earlier.

This is part of a wider trend among young people – towards worsening mental health. In Britain for example, the proportion of fifteen- and sixteen-year-olds who suffer from emotional problems doubled between 1974 and 2004, and it has risen again by 50 per cent since 2004.[12] The problem is especially severe with teenage girls and is heavily focused on anxiety about relationships, appearance and exams. Some 6 per cent of all British children aged eleven to sixteen have

Percentage of students who said 'agree' or 'strongly agree'

	2003	2015	Change
I feel like I belong at school	82	73	-9
Other students seem to like me	85	82	-3
I make friends easily at school	89	78	-11
I don't feel lonely at school	92	85	-7
I don't feel awkward and out of place in my school	90	81	-9
I don't feel like an outsider (or left out of things) at school	93	83	-10

Table 6.1
Fewer children feel comfortable in school (OECD)

tried to harm themselves,[13] and by the age of twenty-four over 18 per cent have self-harmed and over 9 per cent have made a suicide attempt.[14]

Trends in the US are similar. Especially since the spread of social media (see Chapter 13), there has been a huge increase in distress among teenagers in the last few years.[15] How can schools help with these problems?

The purpose of education

We need to start from a clear view of the overall purpose of education. If you accept our Policy Principle, the purpose is simple. It is set out in this box.

> To develop capacities that will increase
> - the happiness of the student (as pupil and adult), and
> - the happiness of the rest of society.

Academic learning is a vital part of this – it illuminates the mind, and it prepares a person to contribute to the rest of society and to earn a living. But children must also learn how to live – how to treat others well and how to manage their own inner life. Education is about drawing out (Latin *educere*) the best in a child, especially the better side of their nature. Various phrases are used to describe these skills of behaving well and being happy. Some call it character, or values; others call it life skills. It clearly goes beyond Grit,[16] and should be a major part of the work of any school. Let us call it wellbeing.

So the wellbeing of the children should be a central goal of school education. Countries vary in what they expect of their schools. In the Netherlands schools are required each year to measure how their students feel about their wellbeing and safety, and this is reported to the Dutch Schools Inspectorate together with a brief account of academic developments in the school.[17] Equally, when private schools in England are inspected, wellbeing (called 'personal development') is now given equal weight with academic progress.[18] But inspectors of the English state schools give it much less importance.

Everywhere, schools are subject to ever more pressure to achieve externally validated exam results. The only way to prevent these exam results from dominating the educational process is also to measure the other things that matter. To improve the wellbeing of our schoolchildren we have to measure it routinely for every child, as they do in the Netherlands.

If you treasure it, measure it

These measurements of wellbeing will serve three functions. They will motivate the school to give more weight to this side of education. They will help prospective parents to know whether their own children will be happy in a school. And they will tell a school which of their children is struggling – something the school does not always know.

It is unlikely that every government would wish to make such measurements compulsory.[19] But once it became more common, it would spread rapidly in response to popular demand, as it has in South Australia.[20] Many suitable questionnaires are available which cover the main things the school needs to know: the children's happiness, their mental health and behaviour, and their experience of the school, including bullying.[21] The questions would be answered both by teachers and (from the age of nine onwards) by the children.[22] Clearly schools differ widely in the kinds of children they take in. So a school should not judge itself by how happy its pupils are, but by whether they become happier as they go through the school (relative to the national average). That should be the key statistic.[23]

So how can schools promote happiness and altruism in their students? It is helpful to look at this under two headings. The first is moral education (the acquisition of values) and the second is specific life skills.

Values

Children absorb moral values from their environment (the ethos of the school) and from specific teaching. Different schools have different approaches. One well-tried method is a code which embodies a set of values. This code is reviewed at intervals through a public debate involving teachers, parents and children; and every teacher, parent and child who enters the school has to sign up to it.[24] The code will influence not just how people behave to each other, but also the content of school assemblies, the truths drawn from many of the subjects taught (like literature), and the content of specific moral education.

The central question in moral education is 'What kind of a person do you want to be?' This can be illuminated from hundreds of role models of noble living, and from the common elements of all the great religions.[25] This topic is surely worthy of at least an hour a week in the school curriculum.

The legal framework for moral education differs between

countries.[26] But no society has flourished unless grown-ups have clear ideas about how one should behave, and transmit them to the younger generation. I believe the central concept should be our Ethical Principle – that we should live so as to increase the happiness in the world (including our own). What an inspiring purpose in life for young people – and so much better than just trying to be smarter and richer than their peers.

Life skills

Apart from values, there are many other specific things which young people need to learn if they are to live well. These include:

- understanding and managing your own emotions ('emotional learning')
- understanding and caring for other people ('social learning')
- healthy living (food, drink, drugs, tobacco, exercise and sleep)
- sexual relationships
- parenting behaviour
- understanding the media
- mental illness and how it can be treated.

Clearly these overlap with values, but they are more heavily empirical – understanding how we are (and not just how we would like to be). In addition there are specific skills, of which the most important is mindfulness. This helps people to calm themselves down and can reduce depression and improve behaviour.[27] It can also improve attention, and thus lead to better exam results.

This set of 'life-skills' can now be taught in an evidence-based way. There are hundreds of brief interventions (twenty hours or less) which have been shown to improve one of the elements in our list of topics.[28] But mostly these results are short-term – one year or less. We can only produce a happiness revolution if these topics are taught continuously throughout the child's school life – with each topic reinforcing what has gone before.

To produce such a continuous curriculum in secondary schools, our research group surveyed all the available short interventions on the topics listed above. We produced a combination which could be taught on a weekly basis from ages eleven to fifteen.[29] This 'Healthy Minds' curriculum has now been tested in twenty-six schools in a randomized trial. The results are highly encouraging. The students had completed detailed wellbeing questionnaires before the course and they did so again four years later. On the primary outcome ('global health') they improved by 10 percentage points, with a similar result for physical health. And on life-satisfaction and behaviour they improved by 7 percentage points.[30] What makes the programme work?

- It does not depend on an inspirational teacher. It consists of detailed materials, and it is the materials which are inspiring.
- The materials focus on good things to do – rather than bad things to avoid. Many 'healthy life' interventions have no effect because they focus on what not to do. If, instead, you have enough good things to do, you will not fill the void with risky behaviour.

- The teachers must be trained to use the materials well.[31] In Healthy Minds it takes five days to train a teacher to use one year's teaching materials. Many of these teachers will teach other subjects. But we also need, in our secondary schools, teachers who have been trained to specialize in teaching wellbeing. These people (often with psychology backgrounds) will become invaluable missionaries for a happy atmosphere in our schools.

The situation in primary schools is different because every teacher will have to teach life skills and be trained to do so. Again, there are successful programmes that have been well researched. For example the PATHS programme (Promoting Attentive Thinking Strategies), which takes up around 130 hours, has been shown to improve behaviour, reduce violence and improve academic attainment.[32]

Positive Education

In recent years Martin Seligman and his colleagues have developed Positive Education as a concept that embraces all that we have been talking about.[33] This movement is flourishing from Australia to Chile, and has spawned its own International Positive Education Network (IPEN). Within this movement, there have been major controlled trials in Bhutan, Mexico and Peru of a fifteen-month wellbeing curriculum in secondary schools, lasting two hours per week. These trials monitored the effects of the curriculum on both wellbeing and academic performance. And does this curriculum help academic performance? It does. In fact, in all three countries, the course affected

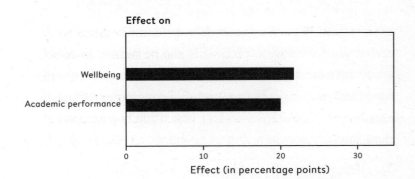

Figure 6.2
Wellbeing teaching improves wellbeing and
academic performance (Bhutan)

wellbeing and academic performance to a similar degree in terms of percentage points.

The results in Bhutan are shown in Figure 6.2. They show that, by the end of the course, the young people who took the wellbeing course had improved both their wellbeing and their academic performance compared with the control group – in each case by around 20 percentage points. Moreover, the gain was still in place a year later. In Peru, the trial involved altogether 700,000 students, using the cascade method: the team trained trainers, who each trained more trainers, who each trained the school teachers. Not surprisingly, the effects on wellbeing and academic performance were smaller (around 8 percentage points), but well worth having. A week-by-week curriculum of positive wellbeing education is now available right through from ages five to eighteen.

Teaching methods and school discipline

Finally, there are the issues of teaching methods and school discipline. There is good evidence that teaching methods send a message to children. If more group-work is involved and less lecturing, children become more trusting and more cooperative in their attitudes.[34] This helps to explain the more pro-social attitudes of Scandinavian adults. Another key issue is the system of motivation. As Carol Dweck has consistently shown, this depends on what teachers praise. If they praise effort, it motivates every student.[35] If they praise performance, it motivates only a few, and for many it results in low mood and feelings of helplessness.

But nothing is likely to work in a school where there is bad discipline. Teachers need to know how to maintain calm and how to look after themselves. One successful approach to classroom control is the famous 'Incredible Years' programme, originally designed for training parents but adapted to training teachers.[36]

As regards the self-preservation of the teachers, one radical approach is for every teacher in a school to become a mindfulness practitioner by taking the eight-week Mindfulness- Based Stress Reduction course (MBSR). This can provide a common culture for a school. It can reduce teacher burnout and bring huge benefits to the children, whether or not the children themselves practise mindfulness.[37]

Much less effective would be a reduction in class size. There is no strong evidence that (with class sizes at their current levels in the West) a reduction in class size improves the happiness of children or their academic attainment.[38] Much better to spend the money on sabbaticals for teachers, better salaries and better training.

Wellbeing in universities

At Yale University the most popular course ever taught is a recent one, 'Psychology and the Good Life'. It gets over a thousand students. This is perhaps not surprising since the President of the university is the psychologist who invented the concept of emotional intelligence. But there are other universities across the world where similar courses are being taught, and in a few it is compulsory (for example, TecMilenio University in Mexico, and the University of Buckingham in Britain).[39]

TecMilenio is a university with 60,000 students across twenty-nine provinces in Mexico. In 2013 its President,

Hector Escamilla, decided to make positive psychology a central ingredient of every student's experience. The aim of the university, he said, should be to help every student discover their purpose in life and then acquire the skills to achieve it. To this end, each student and each staff member has to take a course in positive psychology. For students it is a part of their basic curriculum; for staff it is a digital course taking eighty hours of total study. The university also evaluates policy changes against the criteria of student and staff wellbeing.

Similarly, the Vice Chancellor of the University of Buckingham believes that every university should teach positive psychology to all; they should also offer optional mindfulness classes, give each student a tutor, and a mentor from a previous cohort of students, and regularly measure the wellbeing of every student.[40] But does this approach make sense – and is it enough?

It does make sense, but it is not enough. Centuries ago most university students studied ethics. But not now. Students are preparing for the job market, but what values will they take with them? Surely moral and political philosophy should be standard subjects for every university student. Otherwise what happens? Each adult absorbs the norms of their own profession: economists and businessmen absorb the values of competition; engineers absorb the value of technical excellence; and so on. But where is the ability to assess a situation for its overall effects, and to manage your own conduct accordingly?

I believe that a course which included the philosophy

of the Happiness Principle (plus critiques of it) should be a standard element in university education, together with the basics of positive psychology. If this happened, students could indeed become the standard bearers of the happiness revolution, as they have been of so many revolutions in the past.

Mental health

Going further, educational institutions also have a duty of care for individuals. At some point, at least a quarter of young people will have some mental health problem.[41] Schools and universities need to create an atmosphere where mental health problems can be freely discussed. And they need to know how to refer students for professional help (preferably within their own institution).[42] We shall come to professional help in Chapter 8. But every teacher should have some training in mental health – in how to recognize problems, give students what advice they can, and get them evidence-based professional help when this is needed.

Conclusions

There is no conflict between academic excellence and the acquisition of values, life-skills and happiness. In fact the evidence shows that happier people learn better.[43] And they contribute more to the happiness of the world.

So schools and universities can become society's secret weapon for improving our culture. They already have huge influence on the wellbeing of our children – for good or for ill. But if the effects are to be good, five things are needed:

- Schools must be judged, in large part, by how they promote the happiness and behaviour of their students
- Schools should measure how the happiness of their pupils is progressing.
- The ethos should promote happiness and virtue; students should be non-violent and mindful
- All educational institutions should teach life-skills and values in a fully professional way, and
- They should recognize when students have mental health problems and get them help.

Teachers can do a lot. But when their students eventually go out to work, will their managers offer them an environment which fulfils or disheartens them?

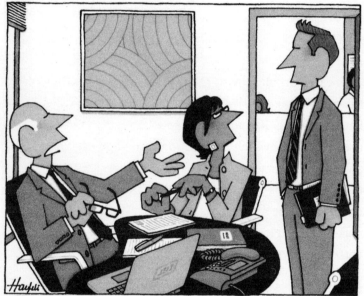

"We want to include you in this decision without letting you affect it."

Managers

> You don't lead by hitting people over the head – that's
> assault, not leadership.
> — Dwight Eisenhower[1]

There is a problem with many line managers – they make the people who work for them miserable. The Nobel Prize laureate Daniel Kahneman has pioneered the study of time-use to find out which times of day are happiest for people, and the answer is quite shocking. As Figure 7.1 shows, the worst time of day is when you are with your boss. The person who should be inspiring you and appreciating your work makes you feel lousy. There must be something deeply wrong with our philosophy of management.

Most work is not enjoyable

There is another, hugely depressing finding that emerges from these studies. Most people don't much like their work – compared with almost anything else they might be doing. Figure 7.2 shows how unhappy people are when they are doing different things. For the average person, working is about the most unpleasant activity there is.[2] This is not of course true for everybody and quite possibly it is not true for many readers of this book. But for the average American citizen it is just that. And the

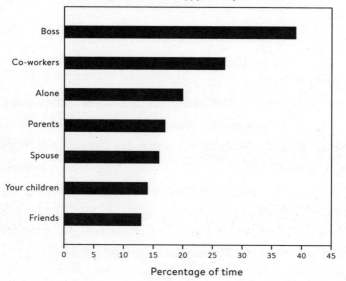

Figure 7.1
Unhappiness depends on who you are with (USA)

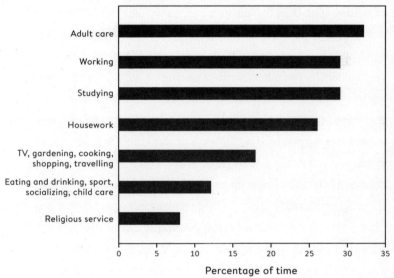

Percentage of time unhappy while doing

Adult care

Working

Studying

Housework

TV, gardening, cooking, shopping, travelling

Eating and drinking, sport, socializing, child care

Religious service

Percentage of time

Figure 7.2
Unhappiness depends on what you are doing

same has been found in Britain. An ingenious app called Mappiness bleeps people at intervals and asks what they are doing and how happy they are.[3] Users of the app are least happy when they are at work – the only thing that is worse is being ill in bed. Moreover, things are not improving and stress is increasing.

But if work is so often unpleasant, one might ask why people are so unhappy if they are unemployed. One reason is of course that they are poorer, but, as we saw in Chapter 2, it is not only that. Work makes you feel needed. Work supplies a purpose in life, a reason to get up in the morning, a sense of being useful – even if it is often boring or hard.[4] It provides a social connection – to other workers and to the customers of your labour – and it provides a sense of meaning and purpose.

But can we produce better ways of working? One thing is obvious: the culture at a workplace is not immutable, nor are the details of how the work is organized or how the workers are paid. If current practice makes people miserable, it can be changed. Even if the job to be done is unappealing, it can be organized in a more appealing and motivating way. Work is not, as the Book of Genesis would have it, a punishment for the sin of Adam.

Happiness and the bottom line

But is it reasonable to expect employers to care about the happiness of their workers? There are two reasons why they should: moral and prudential. The moral reason stems from our Policy Principle: that the objective and *raison d'être* for any organization must be that it contributes to the happiness of the world. This includes the happiness of the shareholders, the customers, the suppliers and the workers (see box below). Contrary to the dogma of many business theorists, it is not only the happiness of the shareholders that should count. Shareholder value has become an increasingly dominant objective in recent years, but all four stakeholders matter,[5] and in English law at least the directors of a company must 'have regard to' the interests of all of them.[6] Profits are essential for a company to survive and grow. But they are not the reason for having companies or for giving them all the protections they receive from the state.[7] Companies exist to serve the interests of all their stakeholders. The workers are generally fewer in number, it is true, than the customers, suppliers and shareholders, but for them it is a much bigger part of their life. So Corporate Social Responsibility starts with the workers.

> The sole purpose of a business is to make the maximum contribution to the combined happiness of
> - customers
> - suppliers
> - shareholders
> - workers.

The second reason for caring about workers is prudential: happy workers work better. Suppose that in 1984 you had invested $1000 in the US companies listed in the 100 Best Places to Work, while your brother invested $1000 in the rest of the market. By 2007 you would have earned $500 more on your investment than your brother did on his.[8] This does not mean that every policy that makes workers happier is good for the bottom line. But it does mean that the happiness of the workers is a serious issue for managers.

This is not surprising since a happier environment attracts and retains better workers.[9] Happy workers are also more productive. This is borne out both by experiment and by observation. So here is a typical laboratory experiment. Two groups of people were given the same specific tasks and paid according to their performance. People who before the task were shown a happy film clip did 12 per cent better than people who were shown a neutral clip.[10] Moreover, happy people tend to do better in their careers. For example, if you take US adults aged twenty-two and follow them up seven years later, those who were happier by one standard deviation when aged twenty-two earn 5 per cent more later (everything else being constant).[11] The weight of evidence supports the conclusion that happy workers generally work better.[12]

What creates a happy workplace?

So what can managers do to improve the happiness of their workers? Needless to say the first step is to have the right people as managers. They need to be appointed as much for their ability to lead as for their technical skills. As the saying goes, 'people don't leave their job; they leave their boss'. But how does a good manager lead?

The basic principles of good work organization are three: autonomy, relatedness, and competence.[13] First, workers need a clear idea of what is expected of them, but also the maximum feasible autonomy in how they discharge their role. Second, they need to feel part of a collective endeavour in which their own contribution is recognized.[14] And, third, they must have the skills and support to do the job – they need to feel competent. The importance of these factors is borne

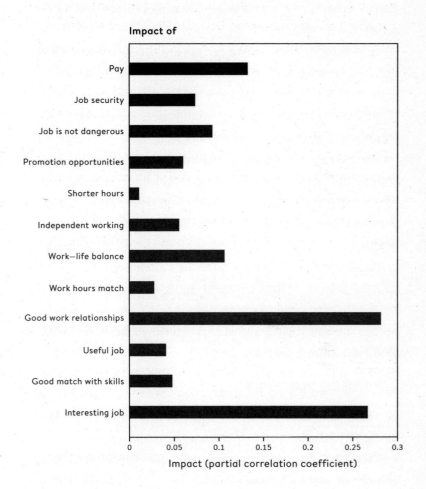

Figure 7.3
How job satisfaction is affected by different aspects of workplace organization

out in Figure 7.3, which comes from the International Social Survey Programme, and assesses what makes workers more satisfied with their job.[15]

In this figure the top five factors are the standard topics of labour market analysis. But the bottom seven are equally important – and they concern the firm's culture and work organization. In particular, they confirm the importance of autonomy (e.g. independent working and work–life balance), relatedness (e.g. good relationships and usefulness),[16] and competence (e.g. good skills match and interesting work). These job-related factors account for nearly as much of the variation in overall happiness as is explained by mental health.[17]

So, how can managers increase the autonomy, relatedness and competence of their workers? For competence, it is pretty obvious – they need to operate good selection procedures, proper training and manageable schedules of work. But what about autonomy and relatedness?

Controlling your work

Workers want a voice in how their work is organized. The STAR initiative was an experiment in providing just that. It was led by a team of American researchers from MIT and elsewhere, and it was designed to:

- give workers more control over their pattern of working hours
- re-orient the culture towards what is achieved rather than how long people are at work
- and encourage supervisors to be more supportive.

Workers met with their team leader and an outside consultant in four two-hour meetings to discuss what changes would work best. And before that the consultant had four hours with the team leader.[18] The initiative was implemented within the IT division of a large US company. Roughly half of the fifty-six working groups in the IT division participated, and the other half (randomly selected) acted as controls.

Six months later the results were striking. As Figure 7.4 shows, job satisfaction increased by 11 percentage points – a major increase. And over the following three years quitting was down by 33 per cent.[19]

One way in which work can become more family-friendly is if it can be done from home. In 62 per cent of all two-parent American households with children, both parents work.[20] So it can be really helpful if one of the parents can work from home. This is not always feasible, but it is possible in many jobs, including call-centre work.[21] So what if call-centre workers are allowed to work from home? Does this produce happier workers and does it improve or damage their performance?

In 2010 a large Chinese travel agency began an experiment to find the answer. They asked all the workers in their Shanghai call-centre (doing airline and hotel bookings) whether they would like to work four days a week from home (and one in the office). Roughly half said yes. Half of those who said yes were then allowed to work at home and the other half (randomly selected) were not. Over the following nine months, those who worked at home reported an 18 per cent increase in life-satisfaction compared with the controls. Their productivity also increased by 13 per cent and their rate of quitting fell

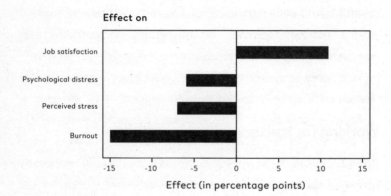

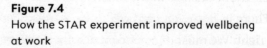

Figure 7.4
How the STAR experiment improved wellbeing
at work

by 50 per cent.[22] The firm was so pleased that it then offered the option of working at home to all of its employees.

These two studies confirm the common-sense conclusion that giving individual workers more autonomy can make them both happier and more productive – a win–win situation.[23] And there should also be higher-level ways of giving workers greater influence at the workplace. The most radical method is making a firm into a cooperative (like the UK's highly successful John Lewis Partnership). Less radical but also worthwhile is having employees as part-owners ('employee share ownership') and having worker representatives on company boards (as in Germany). All of these methods increase workers' sense of autonomy and having a voice.[24]

Working for the team

But what about relatedness? People enjoy being in a team – provided the team works well. But whether teams work well together or become fraught with personal rivalries depends heavily on how the team members are paid.

In 2017 I was speaking to a senior group of HR managers in London. I described in some detail the well-known arguments for paying individuals as precisely as possible for what each of them does – the case expounded so forcefully by many American business schools. And I then said something I had never before said in public: 'Bollocks!' The result was amazing: a massive cheer, followed by a punching of hands in the air. I had said what almost all of them believed but could never say, because it was politically incorrect.

There is, however, considerable evidence that what I said was right. We must of course distinguish between situations where people work in teams and where they work independently – as do sales staff, bond dealers or mechanics when carrying out individual tasks. In the case of independent working, it is natural to pay people by their results. Most studies show that this increases productivity and has no negative effect on life-satisfaction.[25] But what if people are working in teams, as do at least a half of the British workforce?[26] How should each person be paid?

A narrow-spirited view of human nature says that even here we should focus, as best we can, on the individual's contribution to the work of the team. A standard approach is known as 'forced ranking'. In any team the supervisor is forced to rank the members of the team every year; and the bonus each worker gets depends on where they fall in the ranking. The alternative would be to reward all of the team on the basis of the team's performance rather than their own individual ranking. In the narrow-spirited view this team-based approach would provide little incentive, because each individual's effort would make little statistical difference to the average measured performance of the whole team – and thus to his or her pay.

However, the evidence is against the narrow-spirited view. According to data from fourteen American companies and from the US General Social Survey, pay based on team or company performance makes people work harder and quit less often.[27] This is because they are more satisfied with their job. Similarly, in both the European Working Conditions Survey and the British Household Panel Survey, workers who are rewarded for the overall performance of their group or company are more satisfied with their job than other workers.[28] Moreover, a recent study of over 300,000 Danish workers showed that, when performance-related pay was introduced into their company, 6 per cent more of them used anti-depressant or anti-anxiety medication.[29]

But why in the team context does individual performance pay work so much worse than group performance pay? There are two reasons:

1. Individual performance pay produces jealousy
2. Group performance pay enhances team spirit.

Regarding jealousy, people hate to be ranked below others and it demotivates them. Of course, at the same time the people ranked above them may get a boost to their motivation, but this effect is smaller than the first, so that the overall effect on motivation is negative.[30] This has been demonstrated in a number of experiments.[31] In one experiment, a large supplier of office furniture in North America had traditionally ranked all its sales personnel, and then posted the results on its website. But then, as an experiment, it stopped doing this for a randomly chosen group of employees. Over the next two years their sales rose by 11 per cent compared with other workers: they worked better when they were no longer ranked.[32]

It is easy to understand these results because of the negative effect of ranking upon job satisfaction. If you do not know how you are doing relative to others, that ignorance can be bliss compared to knowing and resenting. David Card, at the University of California, Berkeley, did an ingenious test of this.[33] It had recently been decided to put all UC salaries online. But most faculty members did not know that. David Card then randomly informed some of his colleagues at Berkeley that these data were available and measured their job satisfaction before and after doing so, compared with a sample of those he did not inform. Those who had learned about other people's salaries became on average less satisfied. If they earned less than their peers they became less satisfied; and yet if they earned more than their peers they did not become more satisfied. So ignorance was better than knowledge.[34] This must be one reason why a third of American firms make workers sign an agreement not to reveal their remuneration – it would create too much jealousy (and too much pushing for higher wages).

So it is best to avoid regular public rankings of performance. Life, of course, produces its own rankings – periodically some people get promoted while others do not. This is both efficient and inevitable. But we should avoid constant and ceaseless comparison which divides people. Better instead to unite them.

That is what team spirit does, and group-based performance pay enhances team spirit, which in turn enhances performance. Most people like their team to do well, and even people who are not team-players get subjected to peer-group pressure to pull their weight. Moreover, group-based pay reinforces fellow feeling between the members of the group – group loyalty is a powerful motivator. Its power is most evident in war: when soldiers face death in battle, their main driver is loyalty to their colleagues. But group loyalty exists in every well-functioning team. It can be cultivated from the earliest ages onwards. An example of this is the Good Behaviour Game. For the first two years of primary school, the children in a class are split into three teams. Every time a child misbehaves, this is counted as a black mark against the team. Eventually each team is rewarded according to how many times its members have broken the rules. The result is that (compared with controls) the children behave much better; and years later at the age of nineteen to twenty-one they are half as likely to be dependent on drugs or alcohol, or to smoke, or to have anti-social personality disorder, or to have suicidal thoughts.[35] Such is the power of team spirit to have a lasting impact on human behaviour.

I have laboured this point about pay for one very good reason. When I had ended my talk to the HR managers, I asked many of them what action would most to increase the happiness of their workers. Nearly all replied, 'End forced ranking'.[36]

Wellbeing and mental health

Another time, I was chairing the World Economic Forum's Global Agenda Council on Health and Well-being (not as grand as it sounds).[37] We made an important proposal: employers should regularly measure the wellbeing of their workers. Since companies measure other goals, they will only take workers' wellbeing seriously (as a goal) if they measure it as well. There are many good systems of measurement.[38] The results, we proposed, should be published on the front page of every company's annual report.

And we made another suggestion. Managers should be appointed to lead, and an important part of this would be their approach to mental health. Mental illness is a major cost to business. It accounts for a half of all absenteeism, and it also reduces performance on the job – sometimes referred to as presenteeism. Altogether, mental illness reduces the average firm's output by about 2 per cent – leading to a substantial loss of profit.[39]

But of course the worst feature is the worker's own misery; and managers can do a huge amount to reduce this misery. There are at least four steps:

1. First, the manager must recognize that mental illness afflicts about one in seven workers. Managers must have some training in recognizing it and being comfortable talking about it. This means being able to ask, 'Are you OK?'

2. If the answer is 'Not really', the manager has to be able to ask more and discuss what help is available. Many employers have 'employee assistance programmes' which often provide good treatment. But the manager should also know what is available from the health care system at large.

3. If a worker goes off sick, it should be the line manager who calls up and asks what is wrong. It should not be Human Resources. The line manager should care enough about the worker to want to do it.

4. As the person begins to recover, the manager should make it easy for the person to come back to work – part-time if necessary, and sometimes on less demanding work. The key point is that work is a major aid to recovery: once you're ready for it, work is truly therapeutic.

Employers can also play an important role in preventing mental illness arising from whatever cause, at work or outside. They can run courses in, for example, mindfulness or stress management, or (for line managers) on wellbeing-friendly management.[40] Such courses have an increasing evidence-base, which shows that they can improve both mental health and job satisfaction.[41]

Business ethics

These are some of the ways in which employers can improve the wellbeing of their workers. But their responsibilities go wider than this – both to their workers and to their customers. Suppose there is an economic downturn. If it is temporary, companies should (if possible) avoid firing workers, by shortening hours rather than cutting jobs. And if there is a long-term decline in the demand for their products, companies should seriously consider new lines of business in which their workers can continue to be used. Nokia did just that. But if redundancies are unavoidable, companies should (with state help, if necessary) organize retraining and the finding of other jobs.

Business also has duties to its customers. Some companies, including famous banks, sell dud products. Anyone who really believes in the Happiness Principle would not participate in such practices and would if necessary find a different job. More generally, everyone should choose their job so as to make the greatest positive difference to the world (including, of course, their own happiness).

Conclusions

In a capitalist society, most businesses make a big positive difference. And some things are improving. Customer care is hugely better than it was thirty years ago. There is growing concern with worker morale and mental health, and many new consultancies form each week to offer advice on this.

Google offers meditation to all of its workers and prides itself on its happiness Googlegeist.

On the other hand, the old macho culture is still strong – setting worker against worker. The former CEO of General Electric, Jack Welch, practised 'Rank and Yank' – find out who the worst 10 per cent are each year and sack them. This may be less orthodox today, but it is still common. It will require a new generation of managers, believers in the Happiness Principle, to bring a quite different philosophy to the workplace.[42]

If we want a happier society, it is vital that more people should enjoy their work. At present work is, for most people, one of the least happy of all their experiences – worse, for example, than housework. And meeting your boss is the worst time of all. In many firms, the philosophy of management needs to be rethought. This should involve:

- giving workers more influence on how their work is organized
- paying team workers on the basis of team performance
- measuring worker wellbeing
- appointing managers who can inspire and lead
- running courses on wellbeing at work for all their workers
- taking mental illness seriously, with managers who can spot it and get the necessary help.

Firms which do these things will gain both higher productivity and greater profits. And they will make the world happier.

But, if people are mentally ill, what kinds of treatment actually work?

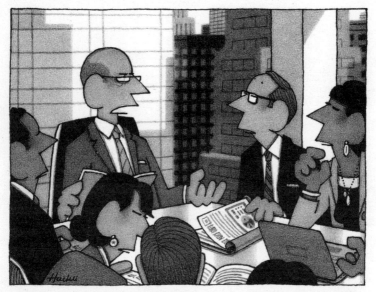

"*Granted it would save countless lives—but to what end?*"

Health Professionals

> Happiness is the highest form of health.
>
> — Dalai Lama

In 1999 Britain established a remarkable institution, with the attractive name of NICE.[1] For every illness, NICE analyses which health care treatments work best – and how much they cost. A good treatment is one which either extends your life or improves its quality or both. To get a single measure of benefit, they add these two effects together into an overall effect on years of life, adjusted for quality. This they call the number of QALYs: Quality-Adjusted Life-Years.

This revolutionary concept was first developed by American academics but, when it was adopted by NICE, it was the first time a government had attempted to measure outcomes in terms of the quality of life as people experience it. Remarkably, QALYs were accepted with little opposition. So NICE was able to assess treatments by the benefit they provided (in terms of QALYs) relative to their cost.[2]

The National Health Service now has the duty of providing – to all who need them – those therapies that NICE recommends. And, broadly speaking, the service does just that for most physical illnesses. But for most problems of mental illness it does not. This is typical of health care worldwide: the shocking failure to give people with mental disorders the well-established treatments that exist.

Ill-health and misery

The failure would not matter so much if mental-health problems were marginal causes of misery. But they are not. In fact, the evidence is that mental illness causes as much misery in the world as is caused by physical illness.

In three advanced countries we can measure mental illness in surveys which ask, 'Have you been diagnosed with depression or an anxiety disorder?' Likewise, we can measure physical illness by the number of illnesses from which people suffer. So how important are mental and physical illness as causes of misery, when compared with each other or with family income (per head) or with unemployment?

To answer this, we first measure misery by looking at a person's life-satisfaction and seeing whether this puts them in the lowest 10 per cent or so in their country. And then we estimate simultaneously the effect of all the four possible causes of why that person is in misery.[3] As Figure 8.1 shows, mental illness is a greater cause of misery than poverty is. And mental illness is also at least as important a source of misery as physical illness is.

In fact, even if we include the poorest countries, mental illness causes at least as much misery as physical illness does.[4] This is because mental illness is not only so devastating when it occurs, but it is also so common. In the typical country about 16 per cent of adults are currently suffering from either depression or from an anxiety disorder such as PTSD (post-traumatic stress disorder) obsessive compulsive

Impact of

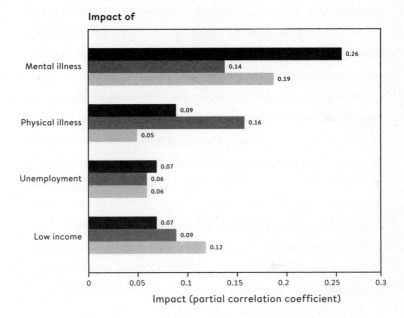

Figure 8.1
How much misery is explained by each factor?

disorder, social phobia, panic attacks or generalized anxiety. In this overall percentage, depression and anxiety are about equally common, but they often overlap. Strikingly, rates of mental illness are similar in rich and poor countries – these problems are not just products of modern civilization.[5] In addition, some 3 per cent of people suffer from severe mental disorders like schizophrenia, bipolar disorder, personality disorders or severe substance abuse.[6]

Mental illness can kill. One way is through suicide – and some 90 per cent of those who will kill themselves are mentally ill.[7] Nearly half of those who commit suicide have suffered from unipolar depression and the rest had even more serious mental illness. In 2013, 840,000 people in the world took their own lives. This was double the number of people who were murdered. And it represented over 1 per cent of all deaths worldwide. By contrast, in the whole of the twentieth century, only 0.7 per cent of all deaths were in battle.[8] Thus in the last century, more people probably died from suicide than in battle.

So mental illness can be deadly serious. Moreover, on top of suicide, mental illness can kill through the effect of the mind on the body. Some of these effects are direct: psychological stress triggers the production of cortisol, increases inflammation and weakens the immune system. Other ways are indirect – via increased smoking, drinking and drug addiction. In consequence, mentally ill people are much more likely to die than others, as Figure 8.2 shows. These deaths are mainly from physical causes, but they also include intentional suicide and accidental suicide through drug overdose, which is now reaching epidemic proportions in the USA.[9]

So is mental illness becoming more common? In Britain

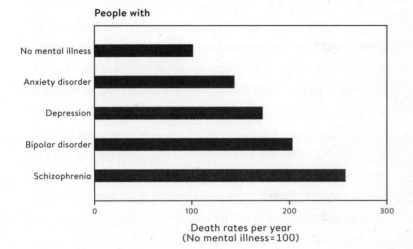

Figure 8.2
Mental illness makes death more likely

and the US it is rising gradually for adults over twenty-five, but more significantly for younger adults, and even more rapidly for adolescents.[10] But, whether mental illness is rising or not, it is one of the worst experiences a person can have. So what can be done about it?

Treating most mental illness costs nothing

The good news is that we now have treatments that can make a real difference.[11] These include many psychological treatments, as we saw in Chapter 3, and also medication. In Britain, NICE recommend medication for all forms of serious mental illness as well as for severe depression and for some forms of anxiety. They also recommend that psychological treatments should be offered for all forms of mental illness. Using psychological therapy the recovery rates for depression and anxiety are at least 50 per cent after an average of about seven sessions, and higher if more sessions are provided. Moreover, such treatments not only reduce people's symptoms but increase their energy and their social connections, which are so crucial to a happy life.

Given the horrible effects of mental illness, one would think that such effective treatments would be at least as available as treatments for most physical conditions. But this is not the case anywhere in the world. In most high-income countries only a quarter of people with depression or anxiety disorders are in any form of treatment,[12] and, more often than not, the only treatment is medication.[13] In the poorest countries the position is even worse, with only one in twenty people being treated.[14]

Common humanity demands that this change. But, sadly,

materialism runs so deep in our culture that what is not immediately visible counts for little compared with suffering which can be seen and touched.[15] So mental health advocates have to deploy another argument – that of economic cost.

Mental illness is mainly a disease of working age, while in rich countries most physical illness afflicts people in retirement. So the economics is quite different for mental illness. One half of all disability in rich countries is due to mental illness, and the same is true of time off work (absenteeism, in the jargon). If we also allow for reduced productivity at work, mental illness reduces the nation's output by about 4 per cent.[16] It also adds to the bill for physical illness, because a person with a given physical illness consumes 50 per cent more physical health care if they are also mentally ill.

For these reasons, there will be massive savings if we can reduce mental illness. The evidence is clear. A programme that provides psychological therapy for depression and anxiety can pay for itself through savings on lost output and on physical health care. And it can help people to a new life.

Improving access to psychological therapy

In 2005 the clinical psychologist David M. Clark and I put precisely these arguments to the British Prime Minister, Tony Blair. At that time, if you had depression or anxiety disorders and sought specialist psychological help from the National Health Service, you would normally be turned down – unless you were a suicide risk or close to that. You might be offered a few sessions of counselling, but not usually of the type recommended by NICE.

And that was the shocking point. NICE were recommending that people should be offered therapy, and it was simply not happening. Moreover, what most of them wanted was therapy – two thirds of people in need say they prefer psychological therapy to drugs.[17] So the National Health Service was not doing its job. Fortunately, the government listened to our argument and in 2008 they launched a new public service known as Improving Access to Psychological Therapies.[18]

To make this succeed, there were three main challenges. The first was to train up a whole new workforce in the therapies that NICE recommended. From 2008 onwards, roughly 1,000 therapists were trained each year. The second challenge was to develop the services within which they should be trained, employed and supervised. By around 2012 there was a service in every area and by 2018 over 600,000 people were being treated annually.

But did they recover? We can only know the answer to that if people's progress is monitored. And it must be done session by session because some people just stop turning up. So the third key feature of the programme was session-by-session monitoring. And from it we learned that, yes, 70 per cent of the people who were treated improved significantly and 50 per cent recovered fully. They had received on average seven sessions. Knowing the outcomes was crucial for the continued political support for the programme.

Of course some local services achieve worse recovery rates than others, and we know a lot about what causes this: too few sessions, less-well-trained therapists, and so on. But one finding is clear: the services that do well are those which use proper diagnostic approaches and provide the right therapy for each patient.[19]

The leading science journal *Nature* has said the service is 'world-beating', and by now a similar approach has been considered – or actually introduced – in at least six other countries.[20] The existing service in England is of course far from perfect. It only treats 10 per cent of all those who are suffering from depression and anxiety. So it needs to become much larger and to offer more sessions. It is only now addressing the huge challenge of helping – in a new way – people who have both a physical illness (like diabetes, angina, lung disease or cancer) and a mental-health problem.

One huge new development is going to be the use of online psychological therapies. These have now been tested successfully in hundreds of trials.[21] They generally work best if linked to some telephone contact with a therapist and should only be used if they are what the patient actually prefers.

One thing is clear. We are dealing here with one of the oldest and largest sources of unhappiness afflicting humankind. Every country will have to tackle the problem in its own way. But in every system there has to be a radical rethinking of priorities. This should not exclude people with severe mental illness. People with schizophrenia or bipolar disorder definitely need medication, but NICE also recommends that they too should get psychological treatment. They ought to get it, and the progress of their mental state should also be routinely monitored.

In rich countries, all the therapy should be provided by specialists – it is the least we can do for people who are in real need. In poorer countries, however, that may not be feasible for some years. The main way forward will be for general health-workers to be given short courses in the recognition

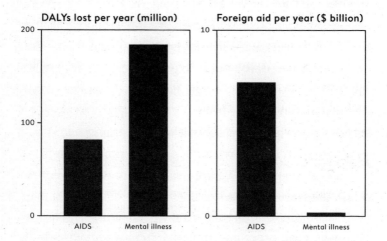

Figure 8.3
Foreign aid discriminates against mental illness

and treatment of common mental-health problems. Trials show this can yield quite good results.[22]

But the scale will have to change everywhere and especially in poor countries, many of which have virtually no mental-health services, even though the problem is as great as in the West. There should also be much more foreign aid allocated to deal with mental health. The worldwide burden of disease (measured by Disability-Adjusted Life Years lost) is twice as great from mental illness as from HIV/AIDs. Yet HIV/AIDs gets roughly sixty-eight times more foreign aid than mental illness does (see Figure 8.3). The attack on HIV/AIDS is vital, but health budgets everywhere need to grow much faster for mental illness than for physical illness. And that is especially so when it comes to children.

Help for children

If a person has a mental-health problem, they need help as early as possible – often in childhood. Over half of the children who have experienced mental-health problems by the age of fifteen will again have mental problems as adults.[23] So why leave treatment until people are adults? By that time, they have felt bad for years. Quite often their education has suffered, and in many cases they have fallen foul of the law – setting them off on a life of constant turmoil.

At any one time, about 10 per cent of children would be diagnosed as mentally ill. Around 5 per cent suffer from some form of anxiety disorder or (less common) depression. And another 5 per cent have serious behavioural problems, sometimes accompanied by ADHD (attention deficit hyperactivity disorder).[24]

But good treatments exist for children as well as adults, though they have been much less well researched. For anxiety and depression, the standard NICE-recommended treatment for children (as for adults) is CBT. For anorexia, it is family therapy. And for behavioural problems, except for the most serious, it is (as we explain in the next chapter) group training of the parent or parents. If the child has ADHD, medication generally helps.

In most countries, most children are not getting the help they need. As with adults, only about a quarter of the children with mental-health problems get specialist help in rich countries, and even fewer elsewhere.[25] In most publicly funded systems, children are only treated if they are incredibly aggressive, or self-hating, or self-destructive. This is a disgrace, and it can only be dealt with in the same way as for adults. A new workforce has to be created, trained in evidence-based therapies, and services have to be created which are easy to access in a non-threatening, informal context. This generally means that they need to be physically based in schools, while being firmly led by health care professionals.[26]

The length of life and the quality of life

I have concentrated heavily on mental health because it is so neglected and has such a major effect on our happiness. But physical health is also vital for our quality of life – and for life itself. This book is mainly about the quality of life. But a good society provides not only happy lives but long ones. As Thomas Jefferson said, the only things that ultimately matter are 'life and happiness'.[27]

So the success of a country depends not only on the

quality of life (and how it varies across people) but also on the length of life (and how that varies across people).[28] In Britain the average length of life is now eighty-two – up from fifty-seven a century ago. That is an amazing improvement. As Figure 8.4 shows, deaths under the age of sixty have largely been eliminated. So there is much less variation than before in how long people live. The variation in the length of life (measured by its standard deviation) is now only fourteen years, compared with twenty-nine years a century ago – an even more incredible improvement and a triumph of modern medicine.[29] Today, we die at much more similar ages than in the past. What a real blessing to couples who love each other.

This change represents a fundamental reduction in health inequality. For the fundamental inequality in our society is the inequality across people and not across social classes. Just as income inequality is across people, so is health inequality.[30] And it is deeply unequal if some people die much younger than others. Fortunately that inequality has been significantly reduced and in fact the length of life is now more equal across people than the distribution of life-satisfaction.[31]

But why has life expectancy risen so much? There are many reasons: higher income, better social conditions, a less polluted environment, and of course modern medicine.[32] Each year medical science becomes better at keeping people alive. But it is much less clever at providing a good quality of life during those extra years. For many patients, the extra years can be horribly painful and humiliating. So there is now a huge debate within medicine about the right balance of effort between improving the quality of life and extending

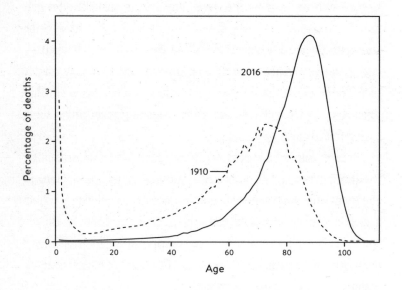

Figure 8.4
Age at which people died in the UK – 1910 compared to 2016.

its length.[33] In England, 15 per cent of all health expenditure goes on the last year of life – which accounts for barely 1 per cent of our total experience of life.[34] In the meantime, there is severe rationing of key expenditures on the quality of life, such as child and adult mental health.

In most cases, sick people really want to go on living as long as possible. But for some people the suffering becomes unbearable and they want to die. If they are terminally ill and want to end it now, we should surely let them do so if they are mentally competent. As autonomous human beings, it should be their right to choose. There should not have to be some grubby underhand arrangement where you have to persuade your doctor to break the law; or, if the docter refuses, you have to starve yourself to death or stop your medication – both of which may have horrible consequences. If people are terminally ill, they should be allowed to die with dignity at a time of their choosing, with their loved ones around them.[35] The US State of Oregon (and now Washington, Vermont and California) allow just that, with strong legal safeguards against unloving relatives applying pressure on vulnerable patients. In twenty years there have been very few problems with this law in Oregon, and it is therefore a model that could be copied worldwide.[36] In Oregon, palliative care has thrived, and the law has brought more openness about dying, and peace of mind to many dying people.[37] The hospice movement, which originally opposed the law, now wholeheartedly supports it.

That said, most of us want to live longer and in better health. Many of us want more health care than we can get. So there is a problem with the existing scale of health care and, as I show in Chapter 11, wellbeing research suggests it should be greater than it is.[38] This is obviously true in poor countries, but it is also true in rich ones. There is also an important and different point about growth over time. It is a universal truth that as people become richer they want more of their money spent on health care. This is because, as incomes increase, the gain in happiness from increased household consumption falls sharply, while the gain from better health care is reduced much less. So in a world where policy is targeted at wellbeing, we ought to see rapidly rising spending on health care.

We should also be doing more to prevent illness before it occurs. Healthy living can be promoted by schools, managers and public health professionals, but it is ultimately a matter for each of us. Like the ancient Romans, we should aspire to 'a healthy mind in a healthy body'. We should sleep properly (preferably eight hours a night), eat well (five portions of fruit and vegetables a day), not smoke, exercise throughout our life, drink responsibly, and take few narcotic drugs.

Narcotic drugs are a health problem

Throughout history, people have sought comfort and joy from mind-altering substances. And, for some people, small doses are not dangerous. The problem is that, for many others, these substances are highly addictive and the results of taking them can be terrible. By far the worst drug is alcohol – about 1 per cent of the population in rich countries become serious alcoholics and of these about one in seven take their own lives.[39] By comparison, natural cannabis is relatively safe, though strong variants can be addictive.[40] Opioids and cocaine, however, are highly addictive.[41]

So should narcotic drugs be banned? The UN's 1961 Single Convention on Narcotic Drugs said just that: it banned all production, sale and use throughout the world. And a few years later US President Richard Nixon declared the 'War on Drugs'.

But this war has been lost. In any Western city today you can find a seller of cannabis, heroin or cocaine within a matter of minutes. But, at the same time, the war has created the biggest criminal industry in human history. The annual turnover is hundreds of billions of dollars.[42] Some of this money has gone to finance terrorism. But, worse than that, the fight for the spoils has generated unparalleled peacetime violence between rival drug gangs, and between the gangs and national security forces. In the rich countries this has filled our prisons to bursting point. And in Latin America more people have died in drug-related violence than in all the violence in Iraq since 2003.[43] It is a total disgrace, for which the rich countries must bear the blame, since they declared the war in the first place and they now generate the profits for the criminals.

So what should be done? Let's begin with the use of drugs, as opposed to their sale. Does it help to make the use of drugs a criminal offence, as the war on drugs requires?[44] Obviously not. People suffering from drug addiction need treatment and they are much less likely to seek it if their addiction constitutes a crime.[45] Instead, they will continue to suffer. They may become thieves to pay for their drugs. Eventually they are likely to get caught anyway, and then receive a criminal record, which makes it even harder for them to earn an honest living. So they keep paying the drug barons, whose profits depend entirely on the illegal nature of the market. It is a totally vicious circle.

So we should decriminalize the use of drugs, making it at most an administrative offence. This is what has been done in Portugal. If you are caught there using drugs, you are sent to a special tribunal which diagnoses your problem. If you are not considered to be addicted, you receive a warning from the tribunal. If you are addicted, you must accept a contract to attend a clinic and, if you do not attend, you get an administrative fine or community service. Most do attend.[46]

Has this more lenient approach increased the problem use of drugs? Not at all. The number of problem users fell when the new system was introduced in Portugal.[47] The Western countries with large numbers of problem users include two of those with the harshest laws: the USA and the UK.[48] Fortunately, however, opinion is changing in both countries – often led by police who are unwilling to waste their time and money on those millions of drug users who cause little trouble.

So, second, what about the sale of drugs? Many drugs such as natural cannabis (not skunk) or ecstasy (MDMA) are less dangerous than alcohol. It is highly preferable that people consume these drugs rather than opiates, cocaine or powerful synthetics. But, if it is illegal to sell any drugs at all, the same gangs will be selling cannabis and hard drugs, and they will push buyers on to the more profitable hard drugs. So we ought to establish a regulated market for relatively safe drugs – as we have done for tobacco and alcohol.

There is another good reason to do this. Most drug deaths occur because people do not know what they are taking. It may be too strong (as ecstasy can be) or it may be adulterated. When the only market for drugs is black, you can never be sure what you are buying. So there is a huge argument for developing a market for the safer drugs that operates in the open, with proper labelling and proper regulation. If such a market were allowed, initially for cannabis and ecstasy, it would displace much of the black market – not only for cannabis but also for the new psychoactive substances and the harder drugs. People would choose the drug that they knew about and that was legal.

But what about the sale of hard drugs? The unregulated supply must remain illegal. But for dangerous substances like heroin, there are demonstrable advantages in the Swiss system of supplying them to addicts for legal consumption in a clinic under supervised conditions.[49] Rational approaches like this will be of huge benefit to people who are addicted and who consume 90 per cent of all heroin. Communities will also benefit. Heroin users who attend clinics reduce their levels of burglary and other property theft by 80 per cent.[50] Fortunately the United Nations, which used to oppose all recreational use of drugs, now accepts a public health approach to drug policy, and countries have been freed to reform their own policies.[51]

There is one other point. Cannabis products have great potential as medicines and as painkillers. For many conditions they are safer and more effective than existing treatments. They provide huge benefits for many patients with epilepsy, multiple sclerosis, chronic neuropathic pain, and nausea/insomnia after chemotherapy.[52] There is an overwhelming case for licensing cannabis products for these conditions. In fact what could be more absurd than allowing opioids to be treated as medicines and refusing to license cannabis products, which are much less dangerous and addictive, have fewer side-effects, and are often as effective? If this were done, millions would benefit.

If we decriminalize drugs and treat addiction as a mental-health problem, we will eventually undermine the giant criminal industry which wreaks havoc on so many continents and fills so many prisons. Cracking the drugs problem is certainly a key element in creating a happier world.

Conclusions

Health is central to wellbeing and, as we become richer, we should give it ever more priority. And this applies in particular to mental health.

- Mental illness causes as much of the world's misery as physical illness does. In rich countries it accounts for more misery than poverty does. Suicide accounts for more deaths worldwide than murder does or (in most years) warfare.
- Good psychological treatments exist, but even in rich countries these only reach a quarter of those in need.
- This is shocking since these treatments pay for themselves. They increase output because more people can work. And they save on physical health care for people with co-morbid physical illnesses.
- In the meantime physical medicine has hugely increased the length of human life and, especially, reduced early death. This is a huge source of increased human wellbeing. But when terminally ill people are in acute pain they should have the choice of an assisted suicide.

- It is vital that narcotic drugs are treated as a mental-health problem and that consumers of drugs are not criminalized. Meanwhile, the sale of unregulated drugs should be a criminal offence, but the safer drugs should be sold (like tobacco and alcohol) in regulated markets.

All health care – physical and mental – attracts idealists. But if you want to fight for a neglected cause, the barricades of today are the barricades of the mind. There can be nothing more challenging or more satisfying than the work of a psychological therapist – to change the course of a person's life.

But shouldn't our parents have made that unnecessary? It is time to examine the role of families.

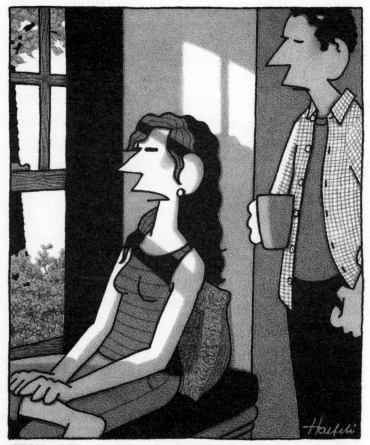

"If I told you where the happy place in my mind is, you'd start showing up there and ruin it."

CHAPTER 9
Families

If you wish for a happy life, you should choose your
parents carefully.
— Michael Rutter and colleagues[1]

'Consider the following statement: Parents getting on well is
one of the most important factors in raising children. Do you
agree?' A British survey posed this question to both teenagers
and parents.[2] Two thirds of the teenagers agreed with the statement, but only one third of the parents did so. As we shall see,
the children were more right than the parents. But how can we
improve our family life and the happiness we get from it?

The family is a complicated business. It is the most basic
of all human institutions. It exists to provide comfort and joy
to adults, and a safe and loving way to bring up children. As
Figure 9.1 shows, many key relationships are involved.

1. There is the relationship between the couple (who may
   or not have children).
2. There are the relationships between each parent and
   child.
3. There are the the way that children affect their parents'
   relationship and the way the parents' relationship affects
   the children – the bit which is so often underestimated
   and yet so crucial.

And there are also the in-laws, grandparents and cousins!

The family

All of these relationships are changing, and patterns of family life have become increasingly varied.

- Most women now go out to work.
- People are marrying later and many choose not to marry at all.[3]
- There is more family break-up than in previous eras.[4] In the past many couples were forced by law to remain in loveless marriages, but now divorce is more widely available. Since women are more able to work and earn a living, breaking up is also more feasible. Nowadays just over 30 per cent of all American children do not live with both their biological parents.[5]
- There has also been a quiet revolution in the way that people find their partners. More and more people find a match on the internet.[6] In 1940 most Americans met their partners through family, school, neighbours or friends.[7] But between 2005 and 2012 one third of US marriages began online. It is encouraging that on average these 'online' marriages proved to be more successful than those made through more traditional routes, both in terms of marital satisfaction and family break-up.[8] But this is still early days for online dating.[9]
- Same-sex couples are now more able to live openly and happily together, and a growing number are starting families themselves.[10]

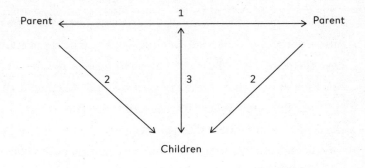

Figure 9.1
The family

- Finally, the relationship between parents and children has changed, with children living in much greater equality with their parents.

Family patterns also differ across cultures. In Latin American countries, for example, family ties are still very strong, which helps to explain why these countries are often happier than others at the same income level.[11] But everywhere change is afoot. So how in this changing environment can we create better relationships within couples, and better relationships between parents and their children? Let's start with the couple.

Loving your partner

I was once at a high-powered conference on the causes of happiness, and over coffee an eminent psychologist took me to one side and said, 'You can list all those things. But the top priority for each of us should be to sustain our feelings for our partner.'

For family conflict is one of the greatest destroyers of happiness both for parents and for children. The parents of course have the possibility of escape – by separation or divorce – and research shows that many couples become happier if they split up. But what is best for the children? This depends on the degree of conflict.[12] If the conflict is bad enough, it is best for the children if the parents separate as amicably as possible, with the children having full access to both parents, preferably on an equal basis. However, if the conflict is not severe, it is best for the children if the couple stay together. And it is best for everybody if the family conflict can be reduced.[13]

But how? Here are two simple psychological approaches which should become widespread in our societies:

1. If conflict occurs, offer Cognitive Behavioural Couple Therapy. This has a good record of reducing conflict.
2. To forestall conflict after the birth of any children, offer ante-natal classes on how to sustain the love between the partners.

These two beacons of hope deserve to be better known, so I will describe how they work in some detail.

If the couple fight

If conflict occurs, the key need is to expand the level of positivity in the relationship. The importance of this has been quantified by John Gottman. He has studied the way couples interact and used this to predict the likelihood of subsequent divorce. If there are more negative interactions than positive ones, this predicts divorce with considerable accuracy.[14]

So how can positivity be achieved? There are now well-evidenced treatments for couples who are unhappy about their relationship – even in cases where there is domestic violence. These treatments ought to be available within any serious health care system.

The best evaluated treatment is Cognitive Behavioural Couple Therapy (CBCT). This has been successfully tested in around two dozen well-controlled trials.[15] It usually involves ten weekly sessions between the therapist and the couple. When they begin treatment, all the couples are distressed about their relationship. But typically, six months after completing treatment, 50 per cent of the couples have become satisfied with their relationship and even five years later the proportion who are happy together is still one third – compared with zero before treatment.[16] Moreover, when one or both partners start off clinically depressed, 57 per cent of them recover during the ten sessions of treatment.[17]

So how exactly does it work? The treatment begins with an assessment of the problem, based on one session with the couple and then a separate session with each partner. From then on, all sessions involve both partners, as well as the therapist. First, they have to agree on the nature of the problem, and to set goals for what they each want from a better relationship. The treatment then aims to produce three types of change, in sequence.

The first is in how the couple **behave** towards each other: how they communicate, how they make decisions, and how they care for each other's needs. The key to communication is listening. So in couple therapy there are periods when couples explicitly talk one at a time – the other doesn't interrupt.

The therapist acts as an impartial controller of the scene, especially when anger and even violence erupt. Partners are often given homework: for example, to write down their view of the problem, or to schedule a structured conversation between themselves on some difficult issue, at a time when they are both likely to be most receptive.

The next set of changes is in how they **understand** each other and themselves. Why did you do what you did? What assumptions are you making about how a relationship should be? Finally, **emotion** trumps all. A partnership only works if people focus on what is good in it. For this to happen, partners can be taught to 'compartmentalize' – to tolerate distressing feelings arising from one part of the relationship, without allowing this to poison all that is good. If you want to express your discontents, you are encouraged to put them in a personal journal.

Going through these steps can transform a relationship. But ultimately of course the message is the same as it is throughout this book:

- We have to behave positively even if the other person doesn't, and
- We must truly imagine what it feels like to be the other person.

So what about **infidelity**? Can a relationship survive that? Often it can, especially with the right help.[18] This involves much longer therapy, usually for six months or more; and both partners must want the relationship to survive. The first step is to confront the pain of the existing situation – to absorb it and to help the grieving process. The next phase is to understand why it happened – why the partner was unfaithful. This should cover both the state of the relationship before the infidelity happened, and the whole background and assumptions of the unfaithful partner. Finally, the stage is reached to move forward – to discuss how the unfaithful partner can make amends and how the injured partner can forgive. Forgiveness here involves a better understanding of the partner – less anger, more compassion and a willingness not to punish.

In some relationships, there is **physical violence**. In fact, about 12 per cent of all partnered men and women in the USA engage in physical aggression, with more extreme violence usually coming from the men.[19] There can also be psychological violence (with or without physical conflict), including extreme withdrawal, denigration or dominance. Intimate partner violence is a major source of unhappiness in every society. It often reflects poor upbringing and chauvinist attitudes which surely need to change at the societal level.[20] But when it does happen, there is a form of CBCT that may be able to provide some help.[21] It focuses specifically on

- the automatic nature of some responses, such as anger, and the beliefs which underpin those responses
- the skills of better communication and problem-solving, and
- the hurt involved in previous fights and other sources of stress.

Couples are typically seen together for fifteen hours in total. But if one partner is a real batterer or if fights continue, the violent partner has to be seen alone. The results of the treatment are usually a reduction in violence and improved satisfaction with the relationship. But equally, if violence continues, the victim needs continued support and the offender needs to be prosecuted.

You might say that couple therapy is simply the wisdom of the ages. Much of it is, but it is arranged so skilfully that people actually accept it and implement it. To deliver basic couple therapy, a therapist who has already had CBT training needs only an intensive one-week course, followed by a year of supervised casework. We should be training thousands of these therapists, since much of the counselling provided today does little more than help people to split up amicably. That is important if the split is inevitable, but we can also do much better at preventing the split.

Preventing family conflict

Ideally we would prevent conflict in the first place. The first major conflict in a relationship often comes when a baby arrives. At that point, most loving couples become less loving: 'satisfaction with the relationship' declines. But this is not inevitable, and it can often be prevented if couples are offered good ante- and post-natal courses that cover not just physical childcare but also the emotional care of the child and of each other. Ideally these courses are free, or nearly so.

In the 1980s Carolyn and Phil Cowan of the University of California at Berkeley developed the following programme. Couples expecting a first child met regularly with three other expectant couples, as well as with a married couple who were psychologically trained and who led the discussion. The meetings ran every week for three months before the birth and for three months after the birth (with all the babies present). The discussion covered essential topics such as how the couple viewed each other; how they talked to each other and solved problems; who did which chores at home; how they planned to bring up the child; which grandparents or relatives would be involved; and how their own childhood experiences influenced their own ideas about parenting.

When the Cowans introduced this intervention as a randomized control trial, the results over the following five years were striking. The couples who had received the extra support remained nearly as satisfied with their relationship as before their child was born. By comparison, the parents who were not given the support became increasingly dissatisfied with their relationship.[22]

In another of the Cowans' programmes, the focus is on how to involve fathers more fully in parenting. In a trial the parents were divided into two groups. In one group both members of the couple came to the meetings; in the other group, only the fathers came. But it was only when the parents came together as a couple that their satisfaction with their own relationship was sustained.[23] The conclusion has to be that couples function best when they discuss their problems together – rather than trying to sort them out on their own.

There are many other programmes for preventing conflict within couples.[24] One of the best is Family Foundations, which involves only eight meetings with the parents (four before the birth and four after). In a randomized trial these parents were followed up three years after taking the programme. Compared with the control group, these parents were less stressed and more cooperative together (by 6 percentage points), and their boys were better behaved and happier (by 26 percentage points).[25] Such programmes should be universally available at little or no cost to the parents. The savings in heartache and social disruption can be massive.

Loving your children

In addition to loving each other, how should parents bring up their children? The basic principles are no longer controversial. First, there must be at least one adult who gives the child their unconditional love. If this happens, most children will automatically form a bond of trust (or **secure attachment**) to the adult(s), which will provide them with a lasting platform of security throughout their life.[26]

This security will be tested by the ups and downs of life, but children should not be artificially protected against minor setbacks.[27] They need to develop **resilience** – the habit of taking a setback as a challenge. This quality can only be developed through learning acceptance and a good philosophy of life.

Next, children need boundaries. They need parents who are **authoritative** and make the boundaries clear – parents who are loving but firm.[28] Children should always be listened to, but three-year-old children do not need to be asked what they want to eat. Parents must stand clearly for certain norms of behaviour. It is only when children are in their teens that parents should want to be on an equal level (of friendship) with their children.

Parents should be hugely **appreciative** of their children, but not in a way that constantly compares them with others – 'you are the greatest'. We do not want to produce narcissists. If we do, those around them will suffer and the narcissists themselves will, in most cases, get their come-uppance.[29]

Children should be mainly praised for effort rather than for achievement. Parents naturally love their children to succeed relative to others, but if children see this, they can easily assume their parents will love them more the more successful they are. This reinforces their competitive instinct and often results in feelings of emptiness and misery. Not all can succeed against others. Instead, we need a **new concept of success,** where we succeed if we use our talents to create as much happiness as we can in the world.

Finally, parents should not feel guilty if their children have problems. Once they have had a second child, most parents realize that every child is different. They differ in their genes.[30] And, in any case, guilt is not a constructive emotion. What children want is love, understanding and care.

Should both parents work?

But who is actually going to do the childcare? And should both parents work? Over the last century, the biggest changes in the world have been the reduction in poverty and disease, and the totally changed role of women. In nineteenth-century families there was an extreme division of labour – with most men working for pay and most mothers working at home (rearing children and caring for the family).[31] Today, women have fewer children, and most women go out to work unless their child is very young. Similarly, men do more of the housework and childcare – but still not generally an equal share on the whole (in Britain eighteen hours a week, compared with thirty-six hours a week for women).[32] The division of labour is changing.

So is it all right for the children if their mothers go out to work? This has been studied repeatedly using naturalistic data on birth cohorts, and there are two general findings.

1. In the first year of the child's life, it is better for the child (emotionally and intellectually) if the mother spends more time at home.[33] So there is a strong case for generous parental leave.[34]

2. After the first year, there is no evidence that, on average, children suffer emotionally or intellectually if their mother spends more time at work. Some individual children may suffer, but in general mothers should relax. If they want a career, the children will usually do fine, especially if working makes their mother happier. To make this possible, there needs to be an effective system of childcare.

But family life is still crucial. Even if the parents work full-time, it is incredibly important that families eat regular meals together. This sharing of experience is one of the surest routes to a happy family life.[35] Each child also needs some quality time with each parent. But what if a child plays up, and you are at your wits' end about what to do?

Children out of control

In 1982 Carolyn Webster-Stratton set up her parenting clinic at the University of Washington in Seattle. Since then she has pioneered the world's most successful treatment for bad behaviour in young children.[36] She does not treat the children directly, but instead she trains their parents – in a programme known as the Incredible Years. In the programme, a group of say ten parents meet with a therapist for two and a half hours a week, over a period of twelve weeks. The typical session begins with a videotape of a parent and child, illustrating which approaches work and which don't.[37]

Webster-Stratton's basic principle is that you get children to behave by appreciating them as much as possible, rather than by making them feel bad. Thus, the early stages of her course teach parents to praise their children as often as possible whenever they do something good. Parents should play with their children, but leave the children to take the initiative at every step. Only later does the course address the setting of boundaries – and finally the issue of consequences. To minimize the sense of grievance, the consequences should be immediate and clearly linked to what has just happened. And the punishment should usually be small, like a five-minute time-out in your room.

Incredible Years illustrates a major theme of this book: we should 'drive out evil with good'. The course has been immensely successful, as shown by numerous controlled trials.[38] In one of these, the children's parents had been trained when the children were aged three to seven and behaving badly. The children were then followed up around ten years later. Compared with the controls, 80 per cent fewer had a diagnosis of serious conduct disorder.[39]

Because of its success, the course has spread worldwide through the 'cascade system'. Mental-health workers can be trained to deliver the course in a three-day training workshop, followed by supervised casework for at least a year. With more training, the trainers can train more trainees and so on. Worldwide there are now 60,000 parent trainers who have been educated in this system. Of course, if children are really difficult they have to be seen and treated directly by a therapist – often with a parent there as well.[40] But with a mixture of psychological insight, scientific method and shrewd organization, Carolyn Webster-Stratton has set an example that can be followed more widely, as we struggle to create happier families and a better world.[41]

Conclusions

The family is the cradle of society. It forms the young, and brings joy and comfort to their parents. But things can easily go wrong – between parents and children, and between the parents themselves. However, modern psychology offers real hope that we can repair these breaches and prevent many of them from happening in the first place.

- If conflict arises, the couple should have access to Cognitive Behavioural Couple Therapy, which will within ten sessions restore over half of all failing relationships.
- When the first child is expected, couples should have access to training on child-rearing and on how to maintain their love for each other. Separate programmes for fathers and mothers are a mistake: they should learn together.
- Children need loving and authoritative parents, who praise their efforts however successful or unsuccessful they are in competitive activities.

- If the children become difficult to manage, one or both parents should go on a course of parent training such as the Incredible Years.
- In the first year after childbirth, there should be generous parental leave. After this, most mothers can safely work, provided decent childcare is available.

However, no family operates in a vacuum. All are based in some local community. So how can communities increase our happiness?

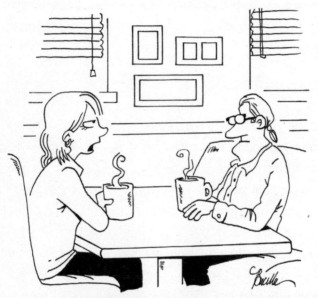

"I'd be more impressed with your hundreds of hours of community service if it weren't court ordered."

Communities

> We have learned to fly the air like birds and swim the sea
> like fish, but we have not learned the simple art of living
> together as brothers.
> — Dr Martin Luther King Jr[1]

At this very moment over one million Britons have not spoken to anyone for over five days.[2] This is deeply shocking. Loneliness is a major problem in modern societies. It is most common in old age, but many younger people also feel it, especially because more and more of them live alone.

In a national survey, British people were asked, 'How lonely do you feel in your daily life?' (on a scale of 0 to 10). As can be seen in Table 10.1, over 15 per cent of all Britons are lonely (answering 6 or above). For old people, loneliness is the biggest single factor affecting their happiness.[3] It also increases their likelihood of suffering from dementia, heart disease, depression, stroke or of death.[4] Being lonely is as bad for your health as smoking is.[5]

Age	
16–64	15%
65–79	15%
80+	29%

Table 10.1
Percentage of people who feel lonely in Britain

The social animal

The reason is that, as Aristotle has said, we are social animals. We need other people for a thousand practical reasons – to eat, procreate, earn a living, and so on. But we also need them for more than that – we need them **for themselves**. We need them for the pleasure of their company. And we need them for the joy of being of use to them – we need to be needed.

As we have seen in Chapter 7, most of us love socializing with people who want our company.[6] It makes us feel understood – that the world is on our side. Moreover, we depend on other people for our own sense of who we are – our identity. Our identity is connected to the kind of people with whom we naturally associate. We can of course choose who we socialize with, but from then on it is a two-way process, as they constantly reinforce our image of ourselves. And that is what gives us the sense of belonging.[7]

We all have multiple identities. We belong to a family, to a workplace, to a group of friends, to a local community, to a country, and even to the world. We can influence each of these groups, and they in turn influence us. In this chapter we shall focus on how our local community affects us and how we contribute to it.

When we associate with people in our community, we usually do it for a particular purpose, as well as for the intrinsic pleasure of being sociable. When adults meet outside the family or work environment, it is generally for one of these purposes:[8]

- eating, drinking, shopping together, or picking up the children
- sports, games and physical activities (e.g. football, gym, bingo, walking, swimming, dancing)
- cultural activities (e.g. religious activities, music, theatre, cinema, arts, libraries, book groups)
- social service activities (e.g. for children, elderly people, sick people, parent–teacher associations, tenants' associations, political activity, professional associations and trades unions).

So who organizes these activities? Many of them are provided by the private sector (like cafés, bars, theatres, cinemas, dancing, yoga classes). Others are typically provided by local government (like swimming pools, libraries and some sports fields). But many are provided by non-profit clubs of all kinds – from golf clubs to churches to social service groups. Let's call them 'community groups'.

These community groups are the heart and soul of many communities, and a key part of the social capital of a society.[9] Some are socially homogeneous (like golf clubs), while others are more socially diverse (like many churches). In the terminology of the great Harvard sociologist Robert D. Putnam, the former provide 'bonding' social capital and the latter provide 'bridging' social capital. Bridging social capital is particularly important for establishing one's general trust in humanity – the importance of feeling that other people are generally on your side.[10] But both types of social capital create the experience of belonging which is so essential for a happy life. And for most people the main sense of belonging still comes from face-to-face interaction rather than from online communities.

So what can be done to increase the sense of belonging to your local community? On the positive side, we can encourage volunteer activity which is the lifeblood of community groups. Planners can also plan the local neighbourhood so that people naturally associate with each other. On the negative side, we have to offer safe and crime-free streets. And we have to construct communities which, however diverse, involve mutual respect and not the feeling of 'them and us'.

Thus in this chapter we will discuss four issues:

1. community groups and voluntary activity
2. crime and the integration of offenders
3. ethnic diversity, and
4. the physical design of cities.

Volunteering

Though many community organizations receive money from the state, they would not exist without voluntary labour.[11] Many are run by volunteer officers and committee members, and nearly all use volunteers to do much of the work on the ground. Voluntary activity on such a scale only happens because it feels worthwhile to the volunteer and, as Chapter 1 showed, there is plenty of evidence that it raises their happiness levels.[12]

Thus voluntary activity, like all giving, is twice blessed – it blesses those that give and those that receive. A good example is the Experience Corps that flourishes in many American cities and enables old people to feel needed by giving meaningful support to children. The volunteers must be at least fifty and they deliver literacy support to primary school children up to the third grade. Most of the volunteers have high school education only, and they get two weeks' training in how to deliver the literacy support. They then work in schools delivering this support for fifteen hours a week. In Baltimore, the volunteers have been carefully followed up in a controlled trial, lasting on average for six months. Compared with a wait-list control group, the volunteers who participated in the trial found they had increased 'the number of people they could turn to for help', as well as their level of physical activity.[13] Over two years, when compared with controls, they were found to have increased their brain volume in both the hippocampal and cortical areas.[14] This makes good sense: contacts between young and old not only help the young, but rejuvenate the old.

Similar principles apply to programmes specifically aimed at reducing loneliness in old age. Many of these schemes save as much as they cost.[15] In one randomized trial in Finland, people were invited into day-care centres where they regularly undertook activities together, including writing, exercise and art. Two years after the initial approach, their subjective health was improved by 25 per cent, and their health care costs were down enough to fully pay for the programme.[16]

Schemes led by volunteers are particularly cheap.[17] In one British experiment, volunteers over fifty-five visited older people who were lonely; they went once a week for ten weeks to help them plan out a more sociable life. In consequence, the old people felt less lonely and developed more social contacts. And the volunteers themselves also felt less lonely.[18]

Volunteering and charity work cannot of course solve all the ills of society – the state also has a crucial role to play. But volunteering widens the network of contacts in a society. As Pope Francis puts it, it involves direct 'engagement' in the lives of others. The opposite is a society where people constantly distinguish between 'them' and 'us' – a society where people have a strong fear or dislike of 'the other'. In the West such 'others' commonly include both criminals and people of different ethnicities. In fact, when Westerners are asked about the problems facing their society, the most commonly mentioned issues include both crime and immigration.[19] Let us take these issues in turn.

Crime and the integration of offenders

Crime affects not only the victims of crime, but also the whole community. For the fear of crime undermines the security of everyone. In Britain, a doubling of the local crime rate reduces the average mental health of the average local resident by 0.1 points (when measured on a scale of 0–10).[20] This is partly because people hugely exaggerate the amount of crime. In one survey 30 per cent of Europeans thought they were likely to be burgled in the next year, whereas in fact the number actually burgled in the previous year was only 1.6 per cent. This discrepancy was greatest in countries with low levels of social trust – countries where general antipathy to 'the other' was at its greatest.[21]

So how are we to reduce crime? One obvious way to reduce reoffending is to stop treating convicted criminals as 'the other'. An impressive example comes from the Singapore Prison experiment. In 1998 the prison service was under enormous pressure. There were high levels of recidivism, and prison officers were leaving in droves due to low morale. But then Chua Chin Kiat was appointed as Director of Prisons. He made each officer responsible for the rehabilitation of a group of prisoners in his block. He gave prisoners a role in the organization of prison life, and improved contacts between prisoners and their families, including tele-visits. He opened prisons to public tours. But, most important, he immediately introduced an after-care system, where care workers whom the prisoners already knew continued to support them after they were released.

There remained the issue of persuading employers to hire the ex-prisoners. So Chua established the Yellow Ribbon Project. It was named after a pop song 'Tie a Yellow Ribbon Round the Old Oak Tree', in which an offender begs his wife to forgive him. In four years some 300,000 Singaporeans participated in Yellow Ribbon activities designed to help ex-offenders. In 2007 and 2009 the Singapore Prison Service was voted one of the best employers in Singapore. It was recruiting with ease. And by 2007 recidivism had fallen from 44 per cent to 26 per cent.[22]

Most people in prison have mental-health problems.[23] They should all be offered psychological therapy and, when necessary, medication. In Washington State, juvenile offenders given Functional Family Therapy by competent therapists were 38 per cent less likely to reoffend over the following eighteen months. And the programme saved much more money than it cost.[24]

But of course it would be best if we could prevent people from offending in the first place. That is the aim of Communities That Care (CTC), a large programme in twenty-four communities across seven US states to prevent problem behaviour by young people aged ten and upwards. The programme does not itself deliver services – it is a system for helping communities to develop the services they need. Specialist trainers hold six training events, roughly one per month in each community, followed by ongoing contacts. When it was trialled, the CTC areas experienced an 18 per cent reduction in youth anti-social behaviour, compared with the matched areas.[25]

Notice that at no point have I talked about criminals getting their just desserts. For that is no part of the philosophy of well-being. As Jeremy Bentham explained over two hundred years ago,[26] punishment can only be justified by its consequences and not because it provides retribution. The consequences that matter are deterrence, protection and rehabilitation:

- punishing an offender can deter him and others from offending in future
- locking up an offender prevents him offending while he is locked up, and
- rehabilitation makes it less likely that he will offend in the future.

Sentencing should be proportional and based on the balance of these three sets of consequences. There is no role for retribution, or 'giving the offender what he deserves'. Retribution is based on a primitive instinct for revenge. But the proper punishment for a crime is the one which produces the best consequences. If the motive is vengeance, the consequences are unlikely to be good. Indeed, even for the victim, it is generally a mistake to suppose that you will be happier if you seek for justice against the perpetrator. Typically this pursuit will simply prolong your agony, often for many years. By contrast, seeking to clarify what actually happened can often help. But eventually the best thing is for the victim to try to accept what has happened, and for society to try to re-establish the offender as one of us.

Ethnic diversity

The same principle of integration applies to people from different ethnic and cultural groups. But it is not easy. In the USA there is overwhelming evidence that people are less likely to trust people from other ethnic backgrounds. And, more than that, in areas of great diversity, people also trust their own sort less, and tend to withdraw from social contacts more generally. And they are less willing to pay for generous welfare benefits and other public goods.[27]

The story is similar in Britain – people are on average less satisfied in areas of mixed ethnicity.[28] However, it seems to have been less true in continental Europe, where there is no long-standing evidence that immigration reduces life-satisfaction. In Germany a careful longitudinal study from 1998 to 2009 showed that people were at least as happy in high immigrant areas as elsewhere (other things being equal).[29] Another study covering roughly the same period, and all European countries, had similar findings when looking at the flow of immigration rather than the stock of immigrants.[30] Looking at the world as a whole, there is no evidence that countries with high proportions of people born elsewhere are, other things being equal, less happy.[31]

Even so, immigration is a highly explosive issue in many countries and has become more so since the wave of migration across the Mediterranean into Europe from 2015 onwards. This is particularly the case for unskilled immigrants, who can sometimes undermine the economic position of native unskilled workers and lead existing residents to move out of their neighbourhoods when the immigrants move in.[32] As we argue in Chapter 11, there must be effective limits to immigration if we are to avoid major social tensions.

But, whatever happens, ethnic diversity will continue to increase worldwide, so how can we make it work for the happiness of all? Many factors are crucial. The first is the law. Laws against racial discrimination and religious hatred have been vital in producing decent, peaceful societies. The second is attitudes – of natives and of immigrants. The Gallup Organization has a measure of how accepting native populations are towards immigrants. And, across the world, both natives and immigrants are happier the more accepting the natives are towards immigrants.[33] Equally, everyone will be happier if immigrants try to assimilate, and this will be easier if they have good access to language classes and to adult education in the ways of their new country. But in the end it is familiarity which breaks down the sense of 'them' and 'us' and turns them into us. So mixed residential areas help and so do mixed schools. There are real problems with schools that cater for children from only one faith or denomination.

Let me end this section with a heart-warming story from India. In 2007 private schools in Delhi were forced to take 20 per cent of their pupils from poor families, who paid no fees.[34] They were also required to integrate the poor students into the same classes as students who were more privileged. The result was a striking change in the attitudes and behaviour of the privileged children. First, they became more inclusive in the friends they made outside school, and in the team-mates they chose at sport. And, second, they became more pro-social – more likely to volunteer for a charity at school and more generous and equitable in their behaviour in laboratory experiments.

Thus it is possible to create real communities from people of very diverse backgrounds – *e pluribus unum* (from many, one). The USA is still struggling with the problem of race relations; many countries struggle with religious and tribal divisions; and the whole world is struggling with immigration. But eventually those who once felt different discover what they have in common; they begin to inter-marry and the differences tend to diminish.

The physical design of cities

Loneliness, crime and diversity are powerful examples of the importance to us of the social context in which we live. But what about the physical context – the layout of our cities, our buildings, our houses, our transport systems and our contact with nature?[35]

In 2014 Britain's All-Party Parliamentary Group on

Wellbeing Economics was taking evidence. Its aim was to investigate how far British policy-making was oriented to the happiness of the people. At one session the group took evidence from a senior official at the Department for Communities and Local Government, the department which regulates the planning system which in turn authorizes the building of new homes.

Planning is a crucial issue in Britain because so few houses are being built that house prices are amongst the highest in the world. One reason for this slow rate of building is the green belt around Britain's major cities: building has not been allowed in these areas, even though much of the land is unattractive and has no public access.[36] This prevents the building of homes in areas where many house-builders are most eager to build them – on the outskirts of our cities. As a result, we have very high rents and house prices. This imposes huge costs on all those looking to rent and on young people trying to buy their first home. It also provides huge gains to the relatively few landowners who are given permission to sell their land to be built on.

So the official was asked, 'How do you think the green belt policy affects the wellbeing of the different sections of society?' He replied, 'You don't understand. The policy is not influenced by wellbeing considerations. It is a simple principle of spatial planning that one community should not expand until it becomes contiguous with another community.'[37]

Fortunately, not all planners and architects think like this, and there is a small but growing number of them who believe in happiness research. Obviously we ought to know how people feel in different environments and, increasingly, we are able to study this – both by asking them and by taking biological measurements as they move around.[38] This should be the basis of the new town planning. This is a massive subject, and here I will discuss only two issues:

1. The provision of opportunities for social connection
2. The importance of green space.

BUILDINGS AND SOCIAL CONNECTIONS

Our buildings, streets and transport systems all have a powerful impact on our experience of our fellow human beings. These processes have been studied over many years, at least since the work of the great urban thinker Jane Jacobs. The central issue is, how close do people want to be to other people if they are to be happy? And the broad answer is: fairly close, but not too close.

We seek a balance, where we can enjoy social exchange but do not have it forced upon us. The majority of humans like a degree of concentrated living (where they can walk to a familiar shopping area or meeting place), but they do not want to be piled on top of each other among hundreds of people they do not know. There is now a significant body of knowledge about how buildings affect people.

- Humans are constructed to walk, and pedestrian areas of the kind pioneered in Copenhagen are a success worldwide.[39]
- People like being with other people and tend to congregate together.[40] The pioneering Danish architect Jan Gehl studied where people sat in a pedestrianized area. More people sat watching other people working on

a building site than sat looking at a shop window or even at a flower bed.[41] People also welcome a reason to slow down, to stop and exchange a word or two.

- People abhor noisy streets, partly because they prevent a civilized conversation. This is one argument for stricter speed restrictions in cities.[42]

- On the ground floors of apartment blocks, people need protective bushes or fences in order not to feel over-exposed.[43]

- In offices and apartment blocks, people abhor busy corridors where unknown people rush past each other.

- In high-rise apartment blocks, people tend to feel isolated as well as crowded in with people they don't know.[44]

- The biggest impact of housing on subjective wellbeing is through its financing and the horrible experience of being behind with your rent or mortgage repayments. In one British survey, no physical aspect of housing (apart from living in a high-rise building) had any detectable influence on subjective wellbeing – neither damp nor overcrowding had any detectable effects.[45]

So town planning is a complicated business, with constant conflicts of interest between different uses of land and between different modes of transport. The ultimate test must be the citizens' happiness. Let us hope that in future architects and planners will study the psychological and physiological responses of potential users of their buildings – before they build them.[46]

GREEN SPACE

One issue is how much land to use as open green space within cities. People are substantially happier if there is green space close to where they live. We can see this from the German socio-economic survey of the same individuals over a long period. Many of these people moved home during the course of the survey and we can therefore see how their happiness was affected by the amount of green space there was near each of their different homes, all else being constant.[47] The data showed that it made a huge difference. If the nearest green open space is 100 metres closer to your home, your life-satisfaction is increased by 0.04 points.

So should we have more green open space in cities? We can begin with two facts. First, if there is an extra hectare of green open space within one kilometre of your house, you are happier by 0.007 points. Second, any hectare in a typical German city is (on average) within one kilometre's distance of 6,000 households. It follows that one extra hectare of green space provides an extra 42 points of life-satisfaction.[48] If the money equivalent of an extra point of life-satisfaction for a year is €150,000,[49] then 42 points of life-satisfaction for a year are worth €6.3 million. In many cities this benefit of €6.3 million would exceed the annual cost of providing an extra hectare of parkland. By contrast, abandoned land close to where people live reduces their happiness – an added reason for turning such space into urban greenery.

But what about the happiness effects of green belts? The same German study showed that happiness was unaffected by how far you lived from the edge of the city.[50] This shows that what people want is parks nearby, not country-side that few will visit – they want green fingers rather than green belts.

Numerous other studies in Britain and elsewhere confirm the positive effects of green space on happiness, on mental and physical health, and on crime.[51] Many years ago Roger Ulrich (then at the University of Delaware) examined the recovery rate from gall bladder operations in a hospital. One group of patients were in rooms that faced trees, and the other group were in rooms that faced a brick wall. The patients who looked out on the trees recovered faster and needed fewer painkillers.[52] Hospital patients also do better when surrounded by pictures of landscapes than when surrounded by abstract art.[53] Crime rates too are lower in greener parts of a city, after controlling for other influences.[54] And, in an interesting lab experiment, people were more generous with their money if they had just been shown slides of nature rather than slides of urban skylines.[55]

One can also see the effects of green space by tracing people's movements day by day. This shows that people feel better in green space than in city streets, and even better when they are in the countryside (though they rarely go there).[56] In one of these studies, people were given wrist cuffs to measure their skin conductance and thus their level of psychological 'arousal'. The study showed that people are much more mellow in green surroundings.[57]

Of course there is nothing like a garden to keep you sane. As they say, 'If you want to be happy for a day have a drink; if you want to be happy for a year have a spouse; and if you want to be happy for a lifetime, have a garden.'

Conclusions

Happiness requires a sense of belonging – not just to your family or your workplace, but also to your local community more generally. You need human contact and it needs to be enjoyable. To make this happen requires good town planning, effective approaches to crime and immigration and great community services.

We need a revitalized local government, committed to raising the wellbeing of its people. Any serious local government will collect data on wellbeing and compare it with benchmarks. It will address the pockets of misery, but all its policies will aim at improving the wellbeing of the people and their sense of local pride and belonging.[58]

We also need thousands of citizens' organizations, running anything from sports grounds to old people's clubs. These organizations cannot exist without volunteers, and the scale of voluntary work is one mark of a happy community. As always, we want the work to be effective, and there is more and more evidence on what really works and what does not.

In these last six chapters we have shown how different groups of citizens can contribute to a happier society. It is time to look at the overall scene, through the eyes of economists and politicians.

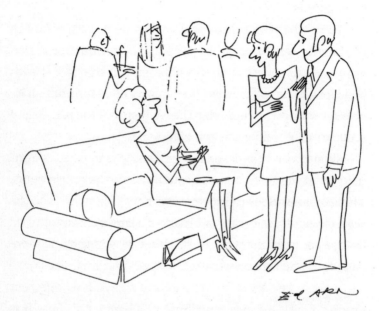

"I'd like you to meet Marty Thorndecker. He's an economist, but he's really very nice."

CHAPTER 11
Economists

> The ultimate purpose of economics, of course, is to
> understand and promote the enhancement of well-being.
> — Ben Bernanke, former Chairman, US Federal Reserve.[1]

When I was twenty-seven, I was appointed as research officer
for a government committee on the future of British higher
education. On my very first day, as I sat at my desk, I was
confronted by a paper from the Treasury. It asked, 'Which
should have the greatest priority: expanding higher education or remaking the decaying cities of the North?' I realized
I had absolutely no way of thinking about this issue; I did not
even know how to begin. The result of this experience was
that I became an economist.

The economic approach

I had discovered that, alone among disciplines, economics
gives us a framework for choosing priorities. This framework
has three elements. First, there is the thing which has to be
maximized – the happiness of the people.[2] Then there are
the constraints – resources, technology and human nature.
And, finally, there are the policy levers – regulations, spending programmes and taxes to pay for them. The challenge is
to choose those policies which produce the most happiness,

while satisfying the constraints. It is a brilliant framework.

The moment I heard about it I bought it. For as a history undergraduate I had read both Jeremy Bentham and John Stuart Mill. They too believed that we should judge the state of a society by the happiness of the people, and I could imagine no better objective than that.

But the next step was trickier. What does happiness depend on? The answer most economists give is, essentially, a person's 'purchasing power' – the mixture of goods, services and leisure that your wage and your unearned income enable you to buy. Since wages and profits add up to gross domestic product (or GDP), this has led to the widespread use of GDP as a measure of the happiness of the people.[3]

When I became an economist, I was quite shocked to discover this practice, because GDP leaves out so much that matters – in fact most of the things that we have discussed in this book.[4] On top of that, it ignores the issue of who gets this money, since it treats a rich person's dollar as of equal value to a poor person's dollar. Happiness research shows how wrong this is: an extra dollar for a poor person produces ten times more extra happiness than an extra dollar in the hands of someone who is ten times richer.[5] But none of this invalidates economics; it just means we have to reform it.

The new cost–benefit analysis

For economics provides us with the vital tool of cost–benefit analysis as the central method of policy evaluation. Cost–benefit analysis makes it possible for us to maximize social wellbeing without Big Brother working out everything in the central committee office. Instead, it relies on individual decision-makers comparing the costs and benefits of every policy, and choosing to do those where the benefits exceed the costs. This works because the costs (properly measured) are the benefits which would follow from the next best use of the same resources. So if the benefits exceed the costs, total benefits increase and so does social wellbeing.[6]

What a wonderful idea. The issue of course is how to measure the costs and benefits. At present the standard approach is to measure costs and benefits in dollars (or in whatever is the local currency). The benefits need not be actual dollars received (like, for example, the extra income due to more job training) – they can also be, for example, the advantage of a bridge which cuts down journey times. In such a case the advantages are measured in terms of the amount of money people would be 'willing to pay' for having the bridge – and this in turn can be inferred from the costs people incur in order to save time in other contexts.[7]

But suppose we want to measure the benefits to society of better mental health, or more stable families, or safer communities, or less unemployment. How on earth could we measure these benefits in terms of the money people are willing to pay for them? There is no plausible way of collecting the relevant evidence, since they are not things upon which people make informed choices based on the observable costs and benefits they bring. They are aspects of life in which people are heavily influenced by things that just happen to them (often from 'outside'). That is precisely why the government has to get involved in them – because voluntary exchange in the market won't produce an efficient outcome.

There are many reasons why markets can fail to be efficient.

There are 'externalities', where one person affects another's welfare not through a voluntary agreement between them but directly. Externalities are pervasive – they include redundancy, the impact of advertising, the experience of crime, and the values we absorb from other people. A second cause of 'market failure' is the existence of public goods, like open space, where charging for use is inefficient. And a third is the existence of information imbalances, where the buyer has no idea of the quality of what the seller is offering. All these factors have huge impacts on human welfare and call for government action. And they make it impossible to measure the benefits of a policy by the money people would be willing to pay for it.

So we need a reformed economics where benefits are measured in units of happiness. Then, if the government has a given sum of money to spend (determined by political forces), it should be spent to produce the greatest additional happiness. This is the policy principle we discussed in Chapter 1. For a policy to be justified, it must produce enough happiness per dollar spent – a sufficient bang for the buck.

Is this way of thinking about policy just pie in the sky? No – something similar has been happening for twenty years in the British National Health Service. The question there is which treatments the service can afford. And the answer is to accept all those treatments which deliver enough improvement in the quality of life relative to the money spent on the treatment – or enough extensions to the length of life itself. Since coherent policy-making requires one single criterion, which includes both the length of life and its quality, the criterion is known as Quality-Adjusted Life Years or QALYs.[8]

There is no reason why a similar approach should not be applied to all public expenditure. Since our concept of the quality of life is 'happiness', a suitable name might be HALYs – Happiness-Adjusted Life Years. Policies would then have to be justified on the basis of their HALYs per dollar.[9] If you object to this criterion, please tell me a better one. For there is currently no overall criterion – just a jumble of incommensurable objectives.

The proposed approach would not supersede existing cost–benefit analysis; it would use the existing framework, but go beyond it. Generally, the impact of policies on happiness would be measured directly (ideally through proper controlled experiments or otherwise through naturalistic evidence). But in other cases the impact would, as now, be measured by 'willingness-to-pay'. But in these cases we should remember that a poor person's dollar produces more happiness than a rich person's. So the estimates of a person's willingness-to-pay should be multiplied by the extra happiness produced per dollar. The result of this calculation is once again a measurement in units of happiness.

Let us be clear. Any cost–benefit analysis which just adds up dollars has no ethical foundation, and this applies to most existing cost–benefit analyses.[10] Instead, we should measure benefits in terms of happiness. These can then be added up across everyone affected or, if the policy-maker chooses, more weight can be given to changes in happiness affecting those whose initial happiness was low. Governments are increasingly interested in using happiness as the criterion for judging policies. New Zealand, France, Sweden, the UK, Bhutan and the United Arab Emirates are all now using it as a criterion (among others).[11] But what difference will this make to actual policy choices?

We have already seen a large number of areas which require more attention and more public money. We want much more spent on people suffering from depression, anxiety disorders, drugs, alcohol and domestic conflict. We need more help for children, for their parents and for their communities. In many cases the extra money will save as much as it costs, through savings on other types of public expenditure, but the cost does need to be incurred in the first place.

Economists should be actively involved in all these areas, because they have the right analytical tools for the job. They are well placed to analyse overall national priorities (that is, which areas need new policies), and then which specific policies are the most cost-effective.

On top of that economists have special expertise in areas traditionally called 'economic'. Among these, I shall only look at those areas where the happiness perspective leads to radically new conclusions about policy priorities:

- economic growth versus economic stability
- low unemployment
- wage inequality, globalization and robots
- the redistribution of income
- world poverty, and
- international migration.

Economic growth versus economic stability

In 2003, the Chicago economist Robert Lucas gave his Presidential Address to the American Economic Association.[12] He argued that economic growth was all-important and that, by comparison, fluctuations in employment mattered very little. If you think income equals happiness, his logic is inescapable – growth at compound interest takes a country to extraordinary heights. But happiness research shows that it is more important for a country to have low unemployment and a stable economy than to have higher long-term growth.

For unemployment is, for most people, one of the worst experiences of life, and as painful on average as being widowed or separated. The loss to the unemployed individual is around 0.7 points of life-satisfaction. On top of this, a high unemployment rate increases the anxiety and insecurity of people in work – they fear for their job and how to get another one if they lose their present one. This spill-over effect quadruples the total loss of happiness when one person is out of work.[13]

People also dislike fluctuations in income. As the Nobel laureate Daniel Kahneman discovered, people hate losing a dollar twice as much as they love gaining a dollar.[14] So economic fluctuations are real destroyers of happiness, and economic stability should be a crucial objective of policy.

Higher long-run economic growth is much less important. There is no conclusive proof that whole societies become happier when they become richer.[15] One problem is that as I get richer, so do most other people – so the norm with which I compare my income rises and my overall happiness rises less than I might have expected.[16] However, governments often think that faster growth will solve their problems with the budget. This is much less true than it might appear. If wages rise, people certainly pay more taxes. But at the same time wages in the public sector have to rise in line with wages in the rest of the economy. So the government has to pay more for a given level of service. This extra expenditure largely cancels out the extra tax receipts.[17] The main advantage to governments from faster long-term growth is that it raises the tax base from which to repay existing government debt.[18] This is a real advantage, but not so important that we should be willing to imperil economic stability for the sake of faster growth.

Unfortunately, that is exactly what happened before 2008. In most countries priority was given to economic growth. The banks argued (wrongly as it turned out) that, if they were less tightly regulated, this would produce higher growth. So governments deregulated the banks as they were asked to. And the rest is history.

Growth is surely desirable and it will happen anyway. It is an aspect of human creativity – we will go on finding better ways to do things as long as humans exist. But faster long-term growth is not an overriding criterion. The leading objectives of macro-economic policy should be stable unemployment and low inflation. In most countries, this is now the job of an independent central bank.

Low unemployment

But unemployment should be more than stable – it should be low. As we said above, unemployment is a prime destroyer of

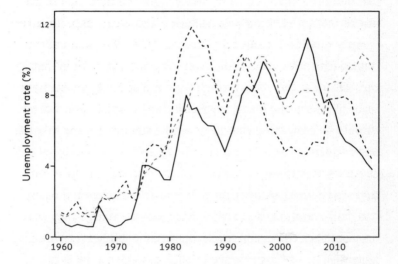

Figure 11.1
Unemployment in Western Europe

—— Germany
--- United Kingdom
--- France

happiness. It makes people feel worthless and unwanted. So when an individual becomes unemployed, the psychic pain is three times greater than the pain from loss of income. And on top of that other people become anxious about their own future, which quadruples the total loss of happiness.[19] So how can unemployment be kept low without the tightness of the labour market creating wage inflation and thus higher prices?

In the 1980s I spent ten years of my life researching this issue with some wonderful colleagues (see My Thanks), and then the next ten years trying to get European governments to implement our ideas. Between the 1960s and the 1980s there was a massive rise in unemployment in most Western countries (see Figure 11.1 above). This was mainly because increased wage pressure had caused high inflation, and then, to reduce the inflation, governments and central banks had deliberately caused higher unemployment. By 1990 inflation was back to normal levels, but unemployment remained high, in spite of the presence by then of large numbers of unfilled job vacancies.[20]

What explained this high level of unemployment when there were still many unfilled vacancies? As our research showed, it was largely due to the system of unemployment benefits. In Europe, benefits were typically available indefinitely and without conditions such as 'you must accept a job if offered'. So, once unemployment had been driven up, many people adjusted to it, however grudgingly. The exception was in countries like Sweden where benefits were less easily available and for a shorter time period; instead, there were active labour market policies to help people back into work – policies like active placement and supported work. So our research concluded that to achieve low unemployment there had to be stricter administration of benefits, linked to more positive help for the unemployed. And, in wage bargaining, it had to be impossible for small groups of insiders to force up the overall wage level.

Since 1990 unemployment has fallen back to its earlier level in some countries but not in others. It has fallen sharply in Germany, Denmark, the Netherlands and Britain, but not in France or Spain. The countries which have done well have indeed introduced stricter conditions for receiving benefits, plus more active labour market policies, and they have avoided wage bargaining systems where small groups of insiders set wages for whole industries.[21] France and Spain have done much less.

But has the lower unemployment actually increased the happiness of those who would otherwise be out of work? The presumption must be yes, but there could be two objections. First, are the extra jobs good enough? The quality of jobs is of course really important. So are we forcing people into bad jobs which are so much worse than their previous job that they would be better off continuing to search? The difference in levels of happiness between the jobs is not large enough for this to be at all likely.[22] Second, some of the jobs are not 'real jobs' but jobs in 'community service', paying little more than unemployment benefit. Can such jobs make people happier than being unemployed? The answer from a number of surveys is yes, people feel much better doing community service jobs than doing nothing at all.[23]

So what is happening? If unemployment is so wretched, why do we have to push people into work. The answer is simple – unemployment can cause not only misery, but help-lessness and despair. Only by getting people active can we help them to overcome despair. That is why a group of us have proposed a radical version of Welfare-to-Work.[24] This requires that every healthy person who has been out of work for over a year should be offered useful activity, paid at the rate for the job. At the same time they should cease to be eligible to claim benefits while being inactive. The principle is, if you like, a right to work linked to a corresponding duty to contribute, in return for income.

In 1997 Tony Blair's government accepted this proposal for people under twenty-five, and the resulting 'New Deal' recovered at least a half of its costs through savings on benefits – paying fewer people for useless inactivity.[25] Then, as youth unemployment fell, the programme became diluted. But in 2009, when unemployment increased again, the government renewed its attack on youth unemployment with a Future Jobs Fund. Again, this recovered about one half of its public cost through savings on unemployment benefits.[26]

Many European countries, influenced by Britain, have followed a similar path: more active help for the unemployed linked to much tighter conditions for receiving unemployment benefits. Denmark was an early mover during the 1990s.[27] But the most striking reforms were the Hartz reforms in Germany beginning in 2003. Though highly controversial, these laid the foundation for Germany's low unemployment in more recent years. One can of course have low unemployment by a fairly draconian system of unemployment relief, as in the US. But a more humane approach to follow is that of Germany or Denmark. Economists in every country need to press for this kind of approach.

One thing that should not be provided is an income guarantee without conditions. Empirically, this reduces the number of people in work, as it has in France. Even worse than that is the idea of a Universal Basic Income, where everyone automatically receives a given basic income whether they need support or not. This is even more expensive than an income guarantee. But both ideas are morally questionable. Income does not just happen: it has to be produced. So if you want a claim on income, you should contribute to the production of it – if you are able to.

Of course there are many people who are not able to work because they are too ill. In a civilized society they are provided with a reasonable income without undue harassment. But governments naturally worry about the cost of these benefits. One approach is to question people closely to see if they really are sick. But a one-off test of 'work capability' is not an adequate way of deciding if they are, because so many illnesses (both mental and physical) fluctuate from week to week in their impact. Terrible misery can be caused if people are tested on a rare good day and subsequently denied benefits. Such crass testing often leads eventually to further incapacity and extra cost. So any test must include a proper medical assessment.

But the best way to reduce the cost of sickness benefits is to reduce the number of people who are sick. In most countries about half of the people on sickness benefit are suffering from mental-health problems, generally depression or anxiety disorders. But typically under half of these people are actually in treatment for their condition, and most of them are on anti-depressants which have clearly not restored them to health. The solution must be that all these people – when they first qualify for benefit – should be given a psychological assessment by a professional therapist and referred for appropriate psychological treatment.[28] Any other approach can lead to real misery.

Wage inequality, globalization and robots

If unemployment is devastating, low relative wages are also demeaning, especially if they are insecure as well. Since the 1980s wage inequality has risen sharply in most English-speaking countries – though little, if at all, in many others (see Table 11.1).

What is causing this new inequality? A common view says it is globalization. And there are obvious examples where employment and wages have been hit hard by foreign competition.[29] However, there is nothing new in this. In the 1950s, 1960s and 1970s Western textiles, steel mills, shipbuilding and consumer electronics were hit successively by competition from emerging countries. Such impacts are severe and they require active labour market policies (including the retraining and placement of displaced workers) and investment subsidies in the towns and cities where the jobs are disappearing. But foreign competition is not the biggest problem: the central issue is technology.[30]

In the sixteenth century Thomas More complained in his work *Utopia* that 'sheep are eating up people'. In the twenty-first century it is machines that are displacing less-skilled workers, while at the same time increasing the demand for

Weekly earnings (90th percentile divided by 10th percentile)

	1980	2010	2016	Change 1980–2016
Australia	2.7	3.6	3.5	+0.7
United Kingdom	2.7	3.7	3.5	+0.9
United States	3.6	5.1	5.5	+1.9
Finland	2.4	2.6	2.6	+0.1
France		3.0	2.9	
Germany		3.3	3.4	
Italy		2.3	2.4	
Japan	2.6	2.9	2.8	+0.2
Sweden	2.0	2.4	2.4	+0.3

Table 11.1
Inequality has risen in some English-speaking countries, but to a
lesser degree elsewhere

people with higher skills. This process inevitably raises the wage premium for skill – unless the supply of skilled workers increases at the same rate as the demand increases. As Table 11.1 implies, the supply of skilled people has not risen fast enough in Britain, the USA or Australia. Although the rate of return to skill acquisition is high,[31] our social institutions have failed to reduce the number of unskilled people fast enough.[32] The result is an ever-greater gap in wages. We are moving towards a two-class society: of graduates (with degrees) and non-graduates (often with few skills). This bi-modal structure of educational achievement is much less evident in continental Europe than it is in Britain or the USA.

So what are the best ways of developing the skills of non-graduates? The main answer is apprenticeship – for many reasons. If you are practically minded, learning makes more sense when you can experience how it is applied, day by day. And if at the same time you earn money, there are powerful motives for learning. The Germanic nations (Germany, Austria, the Netherlands and parts of Switzerland) have the best developed apprenticeship systems. In consequence they have the smallest fraction of young people without skilled qualifications and they have the lowest levels of youth unemployment.[33] So the basic way to reduce wage inequality is to reduce the number of people without a skill.[34] This has always been true, and it will become increasingly important as robots continue to multiply.

However, there is another concern about robots: that they will cause mass unemployment. Is this likely? Economists have always downplayed the fears of technological unemployment. And so far they have always been proved right. After some initial suffering, the weavers found other jobs. So did the horsemen, the ploughmen, the miners, the steel workers and a host of others whose jobs were destroyed by technological advances. Overall, unemployment did not trend upwards, mainly because, when jobs are destroyed and workers are released into the market, new jobs get created. So the overall number of jobs does respond to the number of job-seekers – between 1855 and 2017 the British labour force grew by 168 per cent and, remarkably, so did the number of jobs.[35] There is a market mechanism which increases employment in line with the effective supply of labour. The main issue is at what wage? Robotization will bring downward pressure on the wages of the unskilled, which is why it is so important to reduce the number of unskilled people.

The redistribution of income

But should the state also redistribute money to people with low earning power? Of course it should, for the age-old reason that a dollar transferred from a rich person to a poor one causes more extra pleasure for the poor person than pain to the rich one.[36] Economists have always believed this. At the same time they have usually argued that the size of the pie shrinks as you redistribute the pie. So there is some optimal level of redistribution where the equity case for more redistribution is just offset by the efficiency case against it.[37]

What difference does it make to this argument when we recognize that money has a smaller influence on happiness than economists have tended to assume? The answer is none at all. Even if additional money for the poor will bring them less extra happiness than some have thought, less money for the rich will also cause them less misery than might have been expected.

But there are two new factors coming from the happiness perspective which do introduce massive changes into the redistribution debate. The first makes one more enthusiastic about redistribution. This is the importance of **social comparisons**. As we have seen, people's happiness depends on their relative income as well as their absolute income. So people expend long hours away from the family and friends in order to increase their relative incomes. But for the society as a whole this attempt to raise relative income is a chimera. It can't be done. So what can be done to prevent this source of waste? The answer is simple. When I earn more, I raise the bar against which others compare their income. This makes them worse off. That is a negative 'externality', a form of pollution. And the way to deal with pollution is to tax it. So, up to some level, taxing income improves the efficiency of the economy, by reducing the time wasted on the zero-sum rat race.[38] If this is so, we can obviously undertake more redistribution than we would otherwise, before worrying about its effects on the size of the pie.

But another factor makes one less enthusiastic about redistribution. This is the issue of the **budget constraint.** For practical purposes the proportion of GNP which is raised in taxes has to be taken as given. Money given out to poorer people has to come out of this pot, and we have to think hard about whether money used in this way does more to increase happiness than money provided in direct services aimed at reducing misery.

Is it better to relieve misery by handing out cash or by providing better services? Economists have always preferred redistribution in cash rather than in kind, in the belief that people know more than the state does about what makes them happy. But modern behavioural economics has revealed countless ways in which people's choices are inefficient – they fail to choose what will in fact make them happiest.[39] And they are often desperate for help. So an alternative way to use precious tax receipts is through services which help people to help themselves. The previous chapters have shown many ways in which this can be done. And if we look at the cost-effectiveness of these 'in kind' policies, they frequently do better than simple cash redistribution.[40]

Table 11.2 is a very crude back-of-the-envelope analysis using British data. The issue is, how can we shift people out of misery at the lowest cost? Misery is defined as having life-satisfaction at 3 or below (on a scale of 1–7).[41] From the British Household Panel Study we can then estimate how much money would have to be spent in order to have one less person in misery – depending on the way we go about it. The table suggests that the least efficient of the four options shown is cash redistribution. The most efficient is more money for treating mental illness,[42] and the next most efficient is active labour market policy to reduce unemployment. To devise a more evidence-based multi-pronged strategy for reducing misery is a major challenge which economists need to grasp. Many people believe that household income inequality is the supreme evil, and highlight the correlation between income inequality and poor outcomes to illustrate this.[43] But many of these poor outcomes can be

	£000S per year
Poverty Raising more people above the poverty line	180
Unemployment Reducing unemployment by active labour market policy	30
Physical health Raising more people from the worst 20 per cent of illness	100
Mental health Treating more people for depression and anxiety	10

Table 11.2
Average cost of reducing the numbers of people in misery,
by one person

improved at less cost by direct help, rather than by the further redistribution of income.

For many egalitarians like myself, these findings have come as quite a shock. For many of the happiest countries in the world are the most egalitarian, including those in Scandinavia. And in two compelling books Richard Wilkinson and Kate Pickett have shown a powerful correlation (across countries and across US states) between income inequality and many bad outcomes (including low life expectancy, bad mental health, use of narcotic drugs, crime, teenage pregnancy and the like).[44] So if income inequality 'affects' all these things, one would expect it to affect average happiness as well.[45] Yet in international comparisons, scholars such as John F. Helliwell, who favour equality, have generally failed to pick up an effect of income inequality upon the average happiness of nations, other things being equal.[46]

So what is going on? The answer I suggest is that income inequality has less causal effect on other outcomes than might appear from simple correlation. Instead, both inequality and the other outcomes are jointly determined by a third factor: the spirit of mutual respect in the society. In Scandinavian countries for example there is a strong spirit of mutual respect. This is reflected in good social services which simultaneously improve both the equality of income and all the other outcomes that we value.

This interpretation of the data is supported by a rather remarkable finding. When we compare countries, those with a more equal distribution of *happiness* (rather than of income) are indeed much happier.[47] This too is surely not a causal relationship by itself. But it reflects the fact that, where there is more mutual respect, a multitude of policies are put in place which reduce misery. In addition the general social climate improves. For example, when happiness is more equally distributed, there is more social trust, which benefits everybody.[48] Thus, as Wilkinson and Pickett point out, even the rich have better outcomes in more equal societies. But it is not mainly income equality as such which is producing the greater happiness, but a more general spirit of mutual respect, working through a whole host of channels. This spirit of mutual respect is a key factor affecting the happiness of nations.

World poverty

Up to now our focus has been on the richer economies. But shouldn't priorities be different in the developing world? Not as much as you might think. In poor countries, poverty explains slightly more of the prevailing misery than in rich countries. But even in poor countries there are many other causes of misery beyond poverty and physical illness. Mental illness is at least as big a cause of misery as physical illness is.[49] And in some countries unemployment is another major problem.

Since 1990 there has been a massive fall in world poverty, especially in China. But what has it done for happiness? Among countries for which we have data for fifteen years or more, there is no relation between the rate of economic growth and the change in people's happiness.[50] In fact, in China, the world's most rapidly developing major country, happiness today is little higher than it was in 1990. This is such an astonishing fact that I reproduce Richard Easterlin's graph (Figure 11.2) showing five surveys, all of which tell a consistent tale.

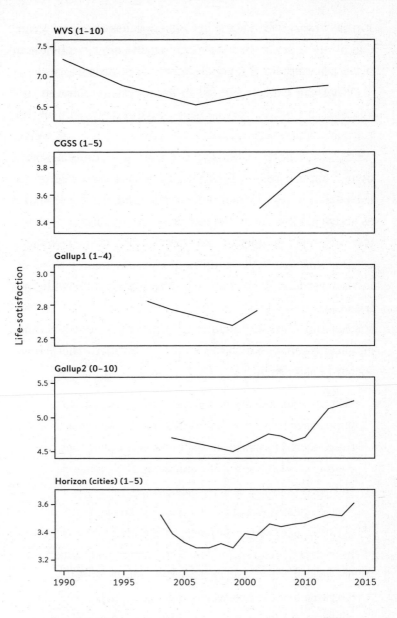

Figure 11.2
Average happiness in China, using five studies, 1990–2015

Virtually every urban home in China now has a colour TV, air conditioning and a washing-machine; and nine in ten have a personal computer. But people appear to be little happier.

What can explain the fall in happiness in China in the 1990s? A part of the story is the massive restructuring of the economy which began at that time. Within a period of twelve years, '50 out of 78 million lost their jobs in traditional state-owned enterprises, and another 20 million were laid off in urban collectives'.[51] Unemployment soared. But so did GDP, as activity shifted from the low productivity factories which were closing, to higher productivity factories which expanded. But this was little comfort to the low-income third of income earners. It was their happiness which fell, while the happiness of the top third was unaffected. And again it was the bottom third who mainly lost the safety net of income and health care to which they had been entitled. This is how Richard Easterlin puts it:

> Why are unemployment and the social safety net so
> important? These two factors bear most directly on
> the concerns foremost in shaping personal happiness –
> income security, family life, and the health of oneself
> and one's family. It is these concerns that are typically
> cited by people worldwide when asked an open-ended
> question as to what is important for their happiness.
> In contrast, broad societal matters such as inequality,
> pollution, political and civil liberties, international
> relations, and the like, which most individuals have little
> ability to influence, are rarely mentioned. Abrupt changes
> in these conditions may affect happiness, but for the most

part, such circumstances are taken as given. The things that matter most are those that take up most people's time day after day, and which they think they have, or should have, some ability to control.[52]

Wise words. But there remains a puzzle. By now unemployment in China has fallen back to its original 1990 level. So why, with all that extra comfort, are people not much happier now than they were in 1990? There are two obvious possibilities. One is that people now use a higher standard of living with which to compare their own – the usual problem of social comparisons. There is some evidence of that.[53] The other is the breaking of social ties. From a static society where people had well-established connections, many have moved to towns in the biggest migration known to man. They miss their social ties and it takes time to develop new ones. So a crucial role of development policy must be to foster real communities in the new urban areas.

In India there are fewer data on wellbeing than in China. But, according to the Gallup World Poll, average life-satisfaction has fallen by 0.7 points (out of 10) since 2008–10 – a dramatic fall.

The challenge to development economists is clear. Grinding poverty has to be eliminated. It destroys happiness and shortens lives.[54] But it is wrong to go for helter-skelter growth. What is needed is a deliberate process whereby genuine communities are maintained or created – communities which give people the feeling of belonging and purpose. It is no easy task.

Is international migration the answer?

Of course, one remedy for world poverty is international migration from poor countries to rich ones. Economists tend to favour migration as a solution, because individuals are likely to increase their income. But what should one conclude about international migration, if wellbeing is what we care about?

The first obvious point is that migration happens because migrants are looking for a better life. And on average they find it. The World Happiness Report for 2018 documents this, using data for over 150 countries.[55] On average, international migrants increase their happiness by 0.6 points (out of 10) – a substantial gain, similar to the gain when an unemployed person finds work.

In fact migrants who move from a less happy country to a happier one become almost as happy as the existing residents in the country where they end up.[56] And surprisingly this happens almost as soon as the migrants arrive. Once they are there, the majority of migrants increase their incomes rapidly, but this does not increase their happiness any further – perhaps because they increasingly compare their incomes with those of other people in their new home country. Similarly the second generation, the children of migrants, are as happy as their parents (perhaps for the same reason) – but much happier than their parents were before they moved.

So why do migrants become happier? It's not just their higher income. Migrants value the social aspects of their society just as much as everyone else does – especially social support, freedom, lack of corruption and generosity.[57] So they become happier mainly because the society they join is nicer – and not only because it is richer.

From the migrant's point of view, their move to another country greatly increases their happiness. But what about the happiness of the two other groups of people affected by the migration? One is the family that the migrants leave behind. According to the evidence, they remain as satisfied with life as before, partly because they often receive money sent back by the migrants (in 2015 the total of such remittances in the world was $500 billion per year).[58]

The other group affected by migration are the people who are already living in the host country. We discussed them in the last chapter. Many gain, but others lose, and hence the issue can become fraught. A decisive factor must be the rate at which immigration occurs. As Paul Collier of the University of Oxford argues powerfully, we cannot have uncontrolled immigration into rich countries. As globalization proceeds and migrant communities in richer countries become larger, there will be ever larger numbers of people wanting to migrate.[59] So there have to be some controls on the rate of annual migration into any rich country.

The optimal level has to reflect the huge potential gains to migrants, but also the legitimate claim of existing residents to determine who comes to live with them.[60] The optimum will surely allow for significant levels of migration, so that as time passes rich countries will become increasingly diverse. But best of all would be a rapid move in the poorer countries towards the wealth and civic standards of the West. This argues the need for a much higher level of foreign aid from richer nations to poor ones.

Conclusions

In conclusion, the economic method is the only way to think about policy priorities: we need to get the most benefit from any money that we spend. But the benefits should be measured in terms of happiness – and not of money. This thinking applies to every issue considered in this book, economic or otherwise. It should apply equally to materialistic projects (like most infrastructure) and to policies with a more social or psychological objective.

The common presumption in favour of physical infrastructure needs to be balanced with a greater concern for the human infrastructure. But the economy does matter, in many ways.

- Economic stability is crucial to our happiness and it is more important than faster long-term growth. We should not imperil stability for the sake of growth.
- Low unemployment is vital and it requires active help to unemployed people to get work. They deserve a right to work within twelve months of becoming unemployed, linked to the ending at that point of unemployment pay for doing nothing.
- Growing inequality is best tackled by providing everyone with a genuine skill (typically through an apprenticeship).
- More cash redistribution may be a less efficient way to reduce misery than many of the ways discussed in earlier chapters.

- Economic development in poor countries should involve a proper balance between increased output and civilized relations at work and in the community.
- International migration brings great increases in happiness to the migrants. But the optimal level of immigration must also allow for the real impact on local residents.
- In all economic decisions there is a major social element that must be considered, for good or ill.

So the happiness approach should become the mainstream method used by economists in the field of public policy. This is now urgent. Behavioural economics has already transformed the way in which many economists explain behaviour. But it requires happiness economics to analyse what types of behaviour are desirable.[61] So happiness economics should become a standard branch of the subject and a standard topic in the economics curriculum.

However, whatever economists advocate, in the end it is politicians who decide. How can they contribute to a happier world?

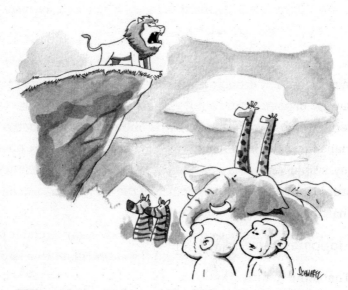

"Did we seriously make this guy the king just because he yells the loudest?"

Politicians and Public Servants

> The care of human life and happiness . . . is the only
> legitimate object of good government.
> — Thomas Jefferson[1]

What should politicians be aiming at? I would, of course, say the happiness of the people.[2] But is that approach going to get them elected? To win elections, what should politicians focus on? According to Bill Clinton, 'It's the economy, stupid.' Well, it's not. A better answer is, 'It's happiness, stupid.' Actually it's both, but happiness is more important than jobs or economic growth.

Happiness affects voting

That's the finding wherever it's been possible to make the comparison. For example, if we take all European elections since the 1970s, the evidence shows that the parties in government get a higher share of the vote when life-satisfaction and economic growth are high. But, as Figure 12.1 shows, more of the variation in the vote is explained by life-satisfaction than by economic growth.[3]

Similarly, if we take all the 3,096 US counties in 2016, the Trump vote in each county is better explained by the average

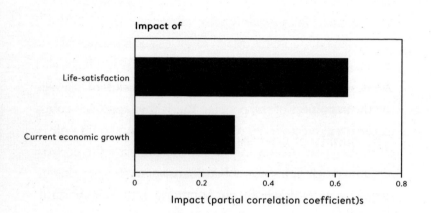

Figure 12.1
Factors explaining the vote share of the existing
government parties (European elections 1970–2014)

happiness in the county than by its unemployment, income or growth rate.[4] There's just more to elections than the economy.

This is very encouraging. So you would think that politicians would be queuing up to learn about the causes of happiness and how to influence it. As we have seen in Chapter 4, some are. But the trickle needs to become a flood. If politicians are looking for a concrete definition of the common good, it is surely encapsulated in the greatest happiness of the people. That is mainly what affects voting. But even if politicians understand this, they still need the evidence on how to increase that happiness. Let's look first at the impact of the quality of government, and then at the issue of the size of government.

The quality of government matters

So how much difference can politicians make to our happiness? As we shall see, a huge difference; and it can be a difference for good or for ill. We need government because so many of our needs can only be satisfied by collective action. We need law and order; defence; the protection of children; the management of health; the enforcement of contracts; the prevention of monopoly; the provision of roads and parks; the regulation of food safety; and so on. It's a long list. Much of it we take for granted, but it is organized by real people. Politicians set the tone, and millions of public servants carry out their policies. The results can be good or bad. Consider, for example, the following incident:

> The minute after she had given birth to her first child
> at one of the public hospitals in the city of Bangalore in

India, Nesam Velankanni wanted the midwife to put the crying baby on her chest. However, before even getting a glimpse of her newborn baby, a nurse whisked the infant away and an attendant asked for a bribe. Nesam Velankanni was told that the customary price if she wanted to hold her child directly after giving birth was 12 USD for a boy and 7 USD if it was a girl. The attendant told her that she wanted the money immediately because the doctors were leaving for the day and wanted their share before going home.[5]

The quality of public services is crucial in any country. So we need good people to go into politics, and in Western democracies we generally get them. I have known many British politicians of various stripes and the majority of them went into politics from an idealistic impulse, even though life as a politician is difficult and constantly exposed to scrutiny. Good politicians need an extraordinary range of skills: good public speaking and debating, good memory, personal charm, decisiveness, thick skin, hard work and good judgement.

It is also important that good people become civil servants, and the evidence shows that civil servants are more public-spirited than the average citizen.[6] Civil servants have immense power and in most cases they affect many more lives than are affected by NGOs. It is a tragedy that public service has lost its appeal for bright young people in so many countries these days. They can generally make at least as much difference through working in the public sector as through working in NGOs.

But where, you may say, is the evidence that the quality of

government makes a difference to our happiness? The World Bank has measured the quality of government under the following two headings:

1. The conduct of the government (including the provision of effective services; a high quality of regulation; the rule of law; and the control of corruption)
2. Democracy (including elections and free speech; and the absence of violence and coups).

Figure 12.2 examines the relationship between the average happiness of a country's population and the conduct of its government. (It covers nearly all countries in the world, but mainly identifies those in the G20.) As you can see, there is quite a close relationship between happiness and the conduct of government and, even if other factors are allowed for, good conduct by the government still increases the happiness of the people.

Moreover, if we look at every country between 2005 and 2012, we find that an improvement of one standard deviation in government conduct increases happiness by at least 0.6 points out of 10.[7] That is a measure of the difference that politicians can make.

It also matters how the government gets appointed. Figure 12.3 shows the crude relation between democracy and the happiness of the people. But, when other influences on happiness are factored in, the impact of democracy is somewhat less clear than the impact of the conduct of government.[8]

However politicians are appointed, they make a huge difference to our lives. When we consider the massive impact

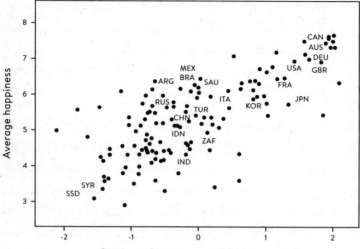

Figure 12.2

Conduct of government (standard deviations from the mean) and average happiness

ARG = Argentina	JPN = Japan
AUS = Australia	KOR = S. Korea
BRA = Brazil	MEX = Mexico
CAN = Canada	RUS = Russia
CHN = China	SAU = Saudi Arabia
DEU = Germany	SSD = S. Sudan
FRA = France	SYR = Syria
GBR = Great Britain	TUR = Turkey
IDN = Indonesia	USA = USA
IND = India	ZAF = South Africa
ITA = Italy	

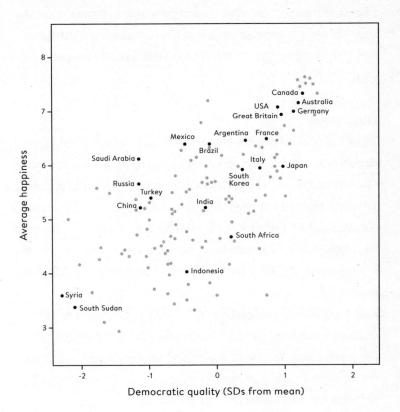

Figure 12.3
Democracy and average happiness (standard deviations from the mean)

ARG = Argentina	JPN = Japan
AUS = Australia	KOR = S. Korea
BRA = Brazil	MEX = Mexico
CAN = Canada	RUS = Russia
CHN = China	SAU = S. Arabia
DEU = Germany	SSD = S. Sudan
FRA = France	SYR = Syria
GBR = Great Britain	TUR = Turkey
IDN = Indonesia	USA = USA
IND = India	ZAF = South Africa
ITA = Italy	

of government on our day-to-day lives, this is hardly surprising. This book cannot be a treatise on good government, but I must make five observations, based partly on personal experience.

LEADERSHIP

Most Cabinet ministers employ, directly or indirectly, thousands (and sometimes millions) of people. So I asked one Cabinet minister, 'Do you think of yourself as leading these people?' His answer was 'No. And I don't know any minister who does.' Instead, their approach is more often to try to manipulate these workers, rather than to inspire them by appealing to their better selves. The result too often is public disillusionment. The great British film-maker David Puttnam, who produced *Chariots of Fire*, was once asked to comment on how British ministers treat their workforces. He replied that Britain was admired internationally more for its army than for anything else, and he had never heard a British general slag off his troops.

So how should a leader lead? Plan long-term: don't just think about the forthcoming year. Imagine where things need to be in five or ten years' time and work back from there. And then transfer that vision to the workforce. The principles of work organization are the same as in business. Set clear goals. Give people as much freedom to deliver them as possible. Support the staff and recognize their achievements.

In every public sector profession the best way to improve performance is through training and retraining – that is more important than all the incentives put together. By updating their skills, people feel competent, stimulated and satisfied.

And the reduced monotony prevents burnout. The world would be a much better place if more energy were devoted to training and less to the next three topics, which typically absorb too much of ministers' time.

REORGANIZATION

Faced with a problem, many leaders will reorganize. A distinguished physician once asked me two questions: which big country has the highest life expectancy and which big country has not reorganized its health care system for over fifty years? The answer to both questions is the same: Japan.[9]

Reorganization of services (and renaming them) is often the least good solution, but is always the easiest to propose if you cannot think of anything else. Any major reorganization totally disrupts the flow of work and creates massive anxiety in the workforce. Frequently the same result could have been achieved by making the existing system work better. A glaring example of this was the disastrous restructuring of England's health service in 2012. Often the best solution involves further training – which would have done much more for the quality of teaching in Britain than all the reorganizations of the last twenty years. When Labour came to power in 1997 its educational mantra was 'standards not structures'. Brilliant. But that was soon forgotten. Interestingly, similar cautions about reorganization often apply to the private sector as well: when one company acquires another its shareholders on average gain nothing.[10] In spite of all of this, people regularly introduce change for the sake of change – who would not want to be called a change-maker? Yet most humans dislike major changes – so shouldn't we take that feeling into account? In every country the majority of people think 'the world today is changing too fast'.[11] We must change what needs to be changed, but we don't have to change everything.

COMPETITION

A common view is that public services suffer from a lack of competition, and therefore new mechanisms must be introduced to make hospital compete with hospital and school with school. This completely ignores the fact that they already compete. There is massive competition within the public service. I did military service in the Royal Artillery and the competition between regiments was ferocious.[12] They competed for reputation. Measuring performance and the benchmarking of outcomes is another healthy source of competition. But material rewards for performance have to be handled with care: natural, healthy competition is good, but 'competition as the be-all-and-end-all' is not. It can easily stand in the way of fruitful collaboration and the sharing of resources, and it can destroy the pleasure of work.

There is another fallacy: that the public sector is inherently less efficient than the private sector. There are in fact classic efficiency reasons why some activities are publicly provided (as well as funded). That said, we have all experienced intense frustration dealing with public sector bureaucrats (in central or local government). But most of us have also had similar experiences dealing with bureaucrats in a private bank or electricity company. It is just not easy to run a user-friendly bureaucracy, especially on a restricted budget. While some services are best provided by the private sector, there are many (including schools, hospitals, social services, prisons and some natural monopolies) where for any given level of funding public provision is at least as good as private.[13]

THE BLAME CULTURE

Government, it is said, must be accountable. That is right. Everything should be out in the open and we should know how our services are performing. But what if they do not perform well? One approach is to say 'heads must roll' and the other is to say 'we must learn from our mistakes'. There are many problems with the 'heads must roll' approach.[14] Inevitably it encourages secrecy: people try to cover up mistakes – the opposite of openness. It encourages the passing of the buck, rather than understanding how each of the many people involved contributed to the mistake.

It also generates a climate of fear. There is a proper level of anxiety appropriate to any important job. But fear is often counter-productive, leading to mistaken priorities. Even when fear is not counter-productive, it is not much fun. And occupations dominated by fear do not attract good people. In 2007, a child known as 'Baby P' died in North London after being tortured by his parents. Many public servants had met this child – doctors, social workers and police. It was a collective failure. But the Secretary of State for Children, Schools and Families decided to sack the head of children's services in the area. His idea was to improve the quality of social services, but the direct consequence of the sacking was that fewer good people went into the profession and many others left it. Social workers became overwhelmed with their caseloads and in the three years after the incident more children were killed by their parents than in the year before 'Baby P' was murdered.[15] Similarly, each time the media force a politician to resign, a life in politics becomes that much less attractive.

There is an alternative to the blame culture. It is to be found in, of all places, the airline industry. Following a terrible air crash in 1978 in Portland, Oregon, the world's airlines introduced what they called a 'just culture'. Their core value is openness and learning from mistakes. So colleagues are encouraged to speak up about what is going wrong. And people who make mistakes are encouraged to acknowledge what they did, without fear of punishment, unless the mistake is intentional or involves gross negligence.[16] Since the system was introduced, the number of airline deaths has fallen from 2 per million passengers in 1980 to 0.01 per million today.[17]

USE OF EXPERT EVIDENCE

In most countries, ministers faced with a problem do not ask, 'Who knows most about this?' They ask, 'Who do we know who knows anything about this?' In his autobiography, Tony Blair was kind enough to say that 'no outside body, no institute or centre of learning' helped him with the policy process 'with the possible exception of the work Richard Layard did for us on the New Deal'.[18] Something is wrong here, and the fault lies with the academics as much as with the politicians. If you want your knowledge to be used, you have to engage with politicians directly and not just with officials. I don't know about other countries, but in Britain anyone can speak to any politician except the Prime Minister by going to a public meeting or a party conference and speaking to them after the event. If more people did this, politicians would be better informed and evidence-based policy would be more common.

Big government?

> Sitting in the dark in his Blackpool bedsit, Harry Harper dialled 999. He told the operator that he had a bread knife at his throat and wanted to kill himself . . . Over six weeks he [had already] visited his local accident and emergency (A&E) unit 28 times . . . 5,000 people attend major A&E units more than 20 times each year . . . Now a promising scheme aims to offer more effective help to the most frequent users, reducing their reliance on emergency services. It was started in 2013 by Rhian Monteith, then a paramedic in Blackpool . . . She asked local NHS managers for the names of the area's most frequently seen patients, and was handed a list of 23 people, including Mr Harper . . . Ms Monteith tried to give them a sense of 'social inclusion and purpose', mentoring them on the phone or over coffee . . . All were given Ms Monteith's phone number and encouraged to call her instead of the emergency services . . . Within months, A&E attendances, 999 calls and hospital admissions all dropped by about 90 per cent among the group . . . The NHS is evaluating the scheme; if it considers it a success, it may be extended nationwide.[19]

So what should the government be responsible for? Before the mid-nineteenth century most Western governments only took responsibility for defence, law and order, poor relief, working conditions, roads and not much else. But then they took on education and health, so that people could become better workers (and soldiers if necessary), and then they took on the macro-economy. These were revolutionary changes in the social order and have played a huge role in the reduction of destitution and disease.

In the next big revolution, the state will help people to become better people – better parents, better partners and saner individuals. That has been the message of this book. The state should offer more help for both mental and physical health, for families in conflict, for addicts, for lonely people and so on. This will not involve more compulsion, nor will it be a nanny state. It will be a state which helps people to help themselves – a state where people take responsibility if they can, but have rights to be helped if they can't.

But how big a state would it be? The policies required are not that expensive and the resulting savings will be substantial. But we must still ask whether people are ready for an increase in the share of national income going on public services and therefore an increase in taxes raised? There are standard economic reasons why they should be. As economic growth proceeds, people are happy to spend a smaller share of total income on material goods like food and clothing, with a rising share going on services. And for many of these services the government is the most efficient and fairest source of funding. For this reason public spending should rise progressively as a share of total national income for many years to come.

In most countries this has happened for much of the post-war period, as Figure 12.4 shows. But in recent years there has been a strong movement to halt the process and even to reduce the share of government spending. The argument

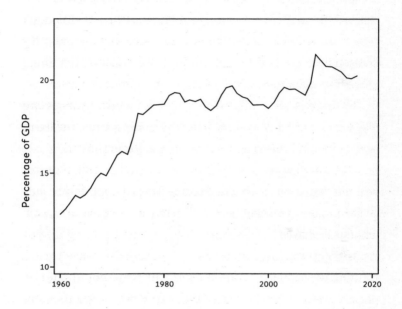

Figure 12.4
Size of government in the OECD (percentage of GDP spent on government goods and services)

has been that people know better how to spend their money than the state does. There is, however, no good evidence that high public spending is bad for economic growth or for people's happiness.[20]

A cross-sectional study of fifteen developed countries addressed the happiness issue. It found that, if a country had increased the share of government services in GDP by 10 points (say from 15 per cent to 25 per cent) average happiness increased by 0.43 points.[21] The study also found a similar effect of welfare spending (relative to GDP) on average happiness.[22]

So there is no evidence that highly taxed countries are less happy on that account.[23] Clearly, citizens value the extra services which the taxes pay for. At the same time the taxes do two other things: they reduce your income (which makes you feel bad), but they also reduce other people's incomes (which makes you feel better).[24] Sacrifice is more tolerable when it is shared.

So a natural question to ask is: can happiness science determine which size of state is best? Not yet, I would say, and possibly never. For the size of the state is a political decision and there are limits to the taxes that people will vote for. By contrast, happiness science tends to favour a much larger state than voters do. This is because of two simple facts: the loss of happiness from taxes is quite small; and the benefits from many types of public service are very large. Let me give an example. Suppose that aggregate tax receipts increase by £15,000 a year, shared across many people. In consequence, the cumulative loss in life-satisfaction is 0.15 points a year.[25] But, if Britain's National Health Service spends this £15,000 a year, it increases life-satisfaction years by roughly sixty times that figure.[26] The ratio of benefit to cost is thus 60:1. This creates a huge presumption in favour of more expenditure, financed by higher taxes.[27] However, it is not realistic to expect the total of public expenditure to be fixed on scientific principles rather than through the political process. The task of policy analysis is, then, as we have shown, to make sure the money is spent in the best possible way. But this becomes more difficult as populism rises.[28]

Why the new populism?

Politics should be informed by reason, fuelled by truth and targeted at the greater good. But recently we have seen huge support for movements which care little about truth and are heavily based on fear of 'the other'. These include the populist anti-immigrant movements in Britain, France, the Netherlands, Italy, Germany, Austria, Hungary, Poland, Denmark and Sweden, as well as the campaigns of Donald Trump and the British Brexiteers. Why have all these movements surged simultaneously?

The usual answer is that more people are discontented than before – due to globalization, immigration and technological change. And it is certainly true that discontented individuals are more likely to vote for populist parties.[29] But is there in fact more discontent overall, or are people simply expressing discontents that have been there for a long time? As the top graph in Figure 12.5 shows, in Western Europe there has been no increase in discontent, at least not in terms of life-satisfaction. The number of people who are not satisfied has fallen, and the number that are satisfied has risen slightly.[30] In Eastern Europe there has been an even more

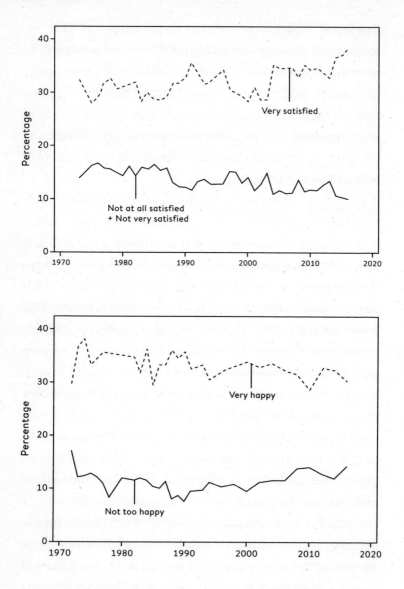

Figure 12.5
(*top*) Life-satisfaction in Western Europe
(*bottom*) Happiness in the United States

marked decline in discontent. Only in the USA is there any evidence of an increase in discontent, but, as the lower graph shows, it is quite modest.

So why are people expressing their sense of discontent more than before? I suggest five factors, all of which have profound implications for the future of our democracies.

THE DECLINE IN DEFERENCE

First, there is the long, secular decline of respect for those in authority. This is in many ways healthy. We should not tug the forelock to kings and queens, nor to head teachers, bishops, judges, pop stars or politicians. Democracy is about equality, and people in authority should earn people's respect rather than assume it. There is, however, one huge long-term problem: the economic troubles of the press and broadcast media lead them to focus ever more on the failures of politicians – and, equally, to underplay the good they do.[31]

Here is some evidence. The graph below (Figure 12.6) shows the balance of news coverage in a sample of news reports from over 130 countries.[32] A more positive value means that on balance the coverage was positive. As is clear, the balance of reporting has shifted strongly in the negative direction. But, as Steven Pinker has argued, the world is not getting worse.[33] So the negative trend is in the reporting and not in the world that is being reported on. This is an ongoing problem, and a major reason for the declining trust in politicians.

HIGH FINANCE AND THE BANKING CRISIS

The second cause of today's populism is more recent, and it is the fault of the politicians. In the two decades before

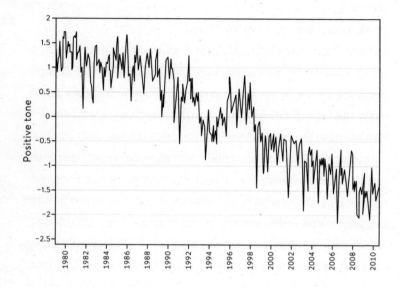

Figure 12.6
Positive tone of the news, 1979–2010

the 2008 financial crisis, politicians in country after country deregulated the banks.[34] The resulting disaster discredited the whole political and business elite worldwide. It showed they did not know what they were doing. Moreover, in the subsequent period of austerity, most bank executives emerged unscathed, while the poor bore the brunt of the cuts.

So what caused the rush to deregulate? There were many factors. There was bad economics, coming largely from US business schools and their finance departments. But the biggest motivation was surely financial. Politicians took money from the banks to finance their political campaigns, and in return they deregulated their benefactors.

Campaign finance is therefore a crucial issue for the future of democracy. Unless political parties become funded mainly by public money, our politics is likely to become increasingly polarized. There will be two opposing groups: an establishment that is increasingly in hock to business, and a populist opposition that grows ever stronger.

SOCIAL MEDIA

A third factor is even more recent: social media. It took off from 2010 onwards and has two important features. First, social media companies have one overriding interest – to keep their clients online and thus exposed to advertisers. And the way to keep people online is to feed them what they like – which means confirming their existing beliefs. In consequence, most people have become more extreme in their beliefs. The recent polarization of American society began with the 1987 law that removed the obligation on the broadcast news to maintain a political balance.[35] But the imbalance has now become much greater due to the way in which social media reinforces people's existing beliefs through what they read – especially if it is 'fake news'.

Equally important is how social media enables people to express these beliefs. It is a curious feature of print that people can express themselves more cruelly and rudely in writing than they ever would do face to face. And social media has now turned everyone into an author. A lot of what is written is incredibly aggressive – the medium (especially when anonymous) has empowered people to express their anger and dissatisfaction more than ever before.[36] No wonder the establishment feels more anxious about the future than for many decades. Social media are now a major institution of society. They bring many blessings, but, as we shall discuss in the next chapter, they can also bring costs. We will have to regulate them, just as we regulate television.

IMMIGRATION

A final trigger has of course been immigration. Immigration into Europe has been much greater than in earlier periods and the year 2015 saw an influx of people across the Mediterranean. The proportion of immigrants in the US population has also risen, though much less sharply than in Europe, and the level is still lower than in 1910. Immigration is experienced by many as a challenge to their own identity, and is a source of anger. Even if it does not necessarily reduce life-satisfaction, it increases dislike of the established elite.

INCREASED STRESS

On top of all this is the general rise in stress that we documented in Chapter 2. As we argued there, this derives from an over-competitive society targeted too heavily on personal success. A better society would produce less populism.

The populism we are seeing is dangerous, and the biggest danger is war. Populists direct the public's anger against a foreign scapegoat and the wars that might follow will destroy happiness.[37] Though war has become less common, that trend could always be reversed.[38] 'Reasonable' people are always amazed at the outbreak of violence. But it corresponds to one basic element in human nature – our tendency to distinguish between 'us' and 'them'. This latent tendency can be triggered by the most trivial of reasons. For example, in one experiment a group of people were divided into two by flipping a coin. Some individuals then had their fingers pricked by a needle, while others watched. Brain measurements showed that the watchers were more disturbed when the person pricked came from their own group.[39] It is this latent tendency to distinguish between 'them and us' that can so suddenly divide people who have lived happily together for centuries – as it did in western Turkey in the 1920s, in Germany in the 1930s, and in Sarajevo in the 1990s. The result is carnage. So, politicians beware. Though demonizing 'the other' is a standard route to short-term popularity, it can ultimately bring disaster to the populists, as it did in Germany in 1945. Politicians should aim at the long-term happiness of their people and not at the empty goal of being better than any other nation. So we must fight the culture of 'them and us' with the culture of compassion.

We have to beat the angry tide of populism. We need brave politicians armed with good policies, who are not in hock to big business; we need much stricter control of social media; and we need a politics of love, not hate.

Conclusions

Barack Obama once said, 'Do we settle for the world as it is, or do we work for the world as it should be?' If you favour the latter, it means working for a happier world.

- If we want a happy society, that has got to be the explicit **objective** of all governments. It is also in their interest, since the happiness of the people is the largest single factor affecting whether the government gets re-elected – even more important than the economy. So, whether they are in power or not, our politicians and our political parties should have the happiness of the people as their goal.

- The **quality** of the government has a huge impact on the happiness of the nation, for good or ill. Good governments provide good services, regulate effectively, control corruption and preserve the rule of law. Ministers responsible for a large workforce should seek to inspire that workforce. They should plan long-term, use evidence from past experience, avoid unnecessary reorganizations, and resist witch-hunts. Power easily corrupts, so we are right to scrutinize our politicians. But this scrutiny, like everything in life, should be sensible. If honest mistakes are allowed to wreck careers, we shall not get good people to go into politics. It is an immensely difficult job, involving inevitable compromise. We should not blame politicians for every compromise or U-turn they make. They should be judged more by the amount of good they do, than by the number of mistakes they make.[40]

- As we become richer, the **size** of government is bound to grow. This applies to the traditional roles of the state, like education and physical health care. But it is also because the public now demand help with mental health, addiction, domestic violence, child abuse and loneliness – not as a nanny state but as a state that helps people to help themselves. Voters will demand that governments provide this type of help, and politicians should adjust their spending plans accordingly. And this will produce a happier world.

- But the big threat for the future is **populism** and the politics of division. We do not want a fractured society. So we have to regulate social media, limit the power of private money in politics and expand state funding of parties. But we also have to address the real concerns that people have in their daily lives.

This requires a new ideology, which concentrates on the things that really matter to people – the things that affect their wellbeing and that of their family, their colleagues and their community. We don't so much need a welfare state as a 'wellbeing state' – one that addresses the needs of all and expects everyone to contribute.

Today, there is massive disenchantment with politics and with the elite. Some people still cling to the ideology of class struggle and others to atomistic versions of liberalism. But most people are ready for a new, more generous ideology which can unite and not divide. This is the ideology of the Happiness Principle and the wellbeing state.

Politicians have a huge responsibility. They set the tone for a society. The laws they pass have huge effects. Politics dominates the news. But people too often complain about what politicians decide, without having themselves engaged in the process. If we want the right things to happen, we have to engage with politicians at every level. There are many ways to improve the human condition and this book has described a number of them. We are all playing different instruments in the orchestra of life, but the conductor is always a politician.

But who is the composer? It is the scientist.

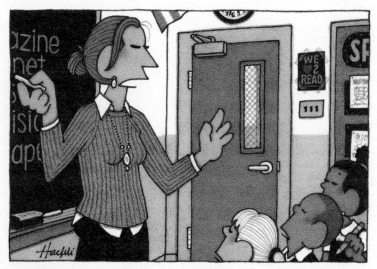

"We capitalize 'Internet' out of respect for its power."

Scientists and Technologists

Knowledge is power.
— Lord Francis Bacon.[1]

Bacon was right. But power to do what? If a young scientist wanted to produce a happier world, what topic would she choose to research?

Clean energy

My number one topic would be clean energy. In 2012, I was sitting on a plane next to the former British Cabinet Secretary Gus O'Donnell and the conversation turned to climate change. Since this is the most urgent problem facing humankind, I asked Gus why there was so little research on cheap clean energy. After all, scientists faced with the Nazi threat had produced the atom bomb within five years. And, faced with the Soviet challenge, they had put a man on the moon in less than ten. If scientists can do these things so quickly, they can surely find ways to produce clean energy that is cheaper than energy from coal, gas and oil.

That is the key to counteracting climate change. Once clean energy becomes cheaper to produce than dirty energy, the coal, oil and gas will simply stay in the ground. International agreements are important for resetting priorities – and regulations, taxes and subsidies help a lot. But the ultimate solution to climate change will be the science of how to produce, store and distribute cheap clean energy.[2]

So what are the scientists up to? Incredibly, until recently only 4 per cent of publicly funded research in the world has been on clean energy.[3] That is all that our governments have been spending on the greatest material problem facing mankind. But, you might say, the private sector can solve this problem – didn't they invent the iPhone? Well, actually, no they didn't. Most of the components of the iPhone were invented through publicly funded research,[4] as were most of the main technological advances of the last hundred years: the computer, semi-conductors, the internet, broadband, satellite communications, genetic sequencing and nuclear power. With clean energy research, as with these other discoveries, the uncertainty and risk is so great that the private sector cannot fund much of the basic work. It needs public money to get many more brilliant scientists to work on these problems.

So, in response to my question, Gus O'Donnell suggested asking David King, who as it happened was going to the same conference as us. David King was the British government's Chief Scientific Adviser under Tony Blair. He, more than almost anyone, was responsible for Britain's pioneering Climate Change Act of 2008, which committed the country by law to progressive reduction of greenhouse gas emissions.[5] In answer to our question, David replied that there was no good reason (except political will) why the world should not double its public spending on clean energy research in a very short time.

Thus was born what became Mission Innovation, a global

commitment in 2015 by the twenty leading countries to double their clean energy research in a coordinated way by 2020. We launched the proposal in 2015, calling it the Global Apollo Programme, to highlight the parallel with the original Apollo moon landing.[6] We also invited the great naturalist David Attenborough to speak at the launch of our proposal. By sheer chance he had been asked a few days earlier to meet with President Obama. Over tea with the President he had commended the proposal, and the President soon gave his support, together with nineteen other leading countries including India and China. It was called Mission Innovation and Bill Gates and other business people also promised $1 billion of private money to follow through on implementing the discoveries made by the programme.

The programme is already well under way.[7] Soon its member countries will be spending $25 billion annually on clean energy research. That is really big money – comparable to what was spent on the original Apollo programme. So now at last we have the money to inspire and energize a whole generation of scientists to work on one of the world's key problems.

The challenge is fascinating and the opportunities immense. For example, the sun provides the earth with 5,000 times more energy than we need. Photovoltaic panels can trap the energy, even when the sun is not shining. The cost of these panels is tumbling, in the same way that the price of computer chips has been falling. Further breakthroughs are also possible using new materials. But then the energy has to be stored for the night-time and for the winter, and a whole range of new storage methods need to be tested. Finally, a new generation of smart grids is needed, as well as electric vehicles and better carbon-free ways of heating and cooling our buildings.

This work is central to the happiness of future generations. If we allow the temperature of the world to reach 2 degrees Celsius above the pre-industrial level, it is likely to stay at that level – or above – for a century or more, because that is how long greenhouse gases stay in the atmosphere.[8] If this happens, there will be major increases in the number of droughts, floods and tempests, leading to mass migration from the worst-affected areas and, inevitably, conflict. Eventually, if that temperature continues long enough, the Greenland ice cap will melt and sea levels will rise by some 7 metres.[9] The climate of the planet, which has been stable since the Stone Age, will be altered – precipitating changes in our living conditions which are very difficult to forecast.

In the face of uncertainty, what do people usually do? They insure themselves. That is the case for action to preserve our current climate. And it is why scientists concerned with human betterment should be flooding into clean energy research.

But sceptics argue that the consequences of climate change are far into the future, and in economic analysis we apply a heavy discount rate to future changes. That may be reasonable if we are talking about future changes in income.[10] For future generations will be richer than we are, and so a loss of income to them will matter less for their happiness than an equal loss of income for us. But when it comes to happiness itself, things are different. Future happiness matters no less than present happiness.[11] And happiness is influenced by much more than income. For example, happiness requires peace and security;[12] and in many areas of the world climate change will imperil both.

The Paris agreement of 2015 went a small way to improve things. But the central forecast is still that the temperature will be an extra 2 degrees higher between 2060 and 2070,[13] and an extra 3 degrees by 2100.[14] So scientists of the world, unite. We need you to save the situation, and to preserve life on earth as we know it.

Science and human need

What else should scientists be working on? And who should decide this? In Britain the decision is made by the scientists and researchers themselves (the so-called Haldane principle). In consequence, decisions about spending resources are mainly driven by curiosity about how life and the universe work. That is a good approach because science so often produces benefits undreamed of by the discoverer. Newton would never have guessed that his principles would produce satellite communications. Like every scientist he was driven by the urge to understand the world.

Even so, it is worth asking how a young scientist wishing to improve human happiness would choose which problems to focus on. In the case of social science the answer is easy. Social science should focus on what causes happiness and misery – both directly and indirectly (through wars, dictatorships and the like). In particular, we now need thousands of controlled experiments (like the few we have described in this book) to discover the most cost-effective ways to improve people's happiness.

When it comes to natural science, I am not qualified to

make detailed suggestions. However, one obvious approach is to ask, 'What are the biggest causes of existing human suffering?' As we have seen, these include:

- pain (physical and mental) and premature death
- poor quality of work.

These are worthy subjects for science in the twenty-first century.

Pain and death

The most obvious triumphs of humanity in recent centuries have been the reduction of physical pain and the extension of human life. Over the twentieth century, average life expectancy in the world rose from forty to seventy years. Most infectious diseases were either eliminated (like smallpox) or dramatically reduced in scale. In rich countries today most people in severe pain (or undergoing surgery) are now treated with painkillers; others buy them at the chemist. It has also become possible to reduce much mental pain with medication or psychological therapy.

Nevertheless, suffering on a large scale continues. Some of this is because of lack of money: we simply do not apply known remedies. But much of it is because we do not know what to do. We have no total cures for most non-communicable diseases (including asthma, arthritis, diabetes, most cancers and many heart conditions). All we have are treatments which ameliorate the conditions. The same is true of schizophrenia, personality disorder, substance abuse, bipolar disorder and many forms of depression. Tackling these problems is a top priority for natural science and, to my mind, more important than improving the productivity of the economy. In fact in the twenty-first century the most valuable aspects of economic growth will be what happens inside our bodies and minds, rather than outside us.

We can only guess at what these advances will be. Our bodies are likely to become full of gadgets (or linked up to them) to make us feel better and live longer.[15] They will also contain replacement parts for different organs. But, more important, we must hope for better ways of treating mental illness – both new psychological treatments and better medication to relieve mental (and physical) pain.[16] Ultimately the body and mind are one; we can help the body by treating the mind, and we can help the mind by treating the body.

Does all this mean that we will become less human? On the contrary, we will be more like we want to be. Most people on antidepressants report that they are now more like their 'real selves', not less so.[17]

But we cannot avoid two big problems resulting from our success. The first is the suffering caused by our enhanced ability to preserve life, but at very low quality. If people in terrible pain want to die, they should be allowed to undertake an assisted suicide, subject to strict legal safeguards – as we argued in Chapter 8. Equally, if parents want to preserve a severely premature baby for a life of unbearable suffering, doctors need the right to say No, on behalf of the child.[18] The second problem is the pressure on medicine to enhance our capacities positively, as well as to reduce our suffering. We reject doping in sport. But should we also reject cognitive enhancers or aids to physical activity or positive living?

If there are no bad side-effects, I cannot see why we should object to any of this.

A more extreme question is this. Suppose we could use DNA to predict a person's probability of happiness, which we can already do with some degree of accuracy.[19] Should we allow doctors to offer in vitro fertilization for, say, four eggs and then choose the best embryo (with, for example, the DNA predisposed for the greatest happiness)? I suspect that eventually it will happen.[20] The most obvious danger is that parents will select on grounds of sex, producing an imbalance of sexes in the population.

Artificial intelligence and robots

What about work? As we have seen, most people enjoy their job less than they enjoy most other things, including housework. This is a disturbing fact about rich countries. Equally, in poor countries many people undertake back-breaking toil, in which their feelings are numbed by exhaustion for much of the time. So should we welcome AI and robots?

Artificial intelligence will certainly displace some mental activities that are quite interesting: for example, much medical diagnosis. But robots will mainly replace drudgery – routine activities, physical or mental. As we argued in Chapter 11, this will not cause an upward trend in unemployment. It will of course cause massive changes in the structure of employment. But this is what has happened throughout modern history: looms replaced weavers; tractors and cars replaced horsemen; washing machines replaced laundrywomen; and so on. Yet no upward trend in unemployment resulted. The changes were hard on those affected, and many of them had long spells out of work. But, despite massive population increases over two centuries, the unemployment rate has not risen. This is because the labour market operates like other markets, and (apart from structural impediments) the workers seeking work get hired – at some wage or other.[21] The main issue for the future is at what wage. Clearly, AI and robotics will increase the demand for technologists, whose real wages will rise. And they will reduce the demand for less skilled people, whose real wages will fall, unless their supply falls even faster. These trends make better education for the less able students even more crucial.

What about hours of work? AI and robotization are likely to raise the average wage. In consequence we can expect average hours of work to fall, as people choose more leisure. But how will they spend their leisure time? They will enjoy it a lot more if they have had a broad education, which includes music, dance, drama and art. In the age of robotics, there is no case for a productivity-above-all-things system of education. As people become less preoccupied with money, they will only be happy when they find other purposes in life – either social or aesthetic.

Social media and data

Not all technology is unambiguously good and this applies particularly to social media. Here the positive potential is clear, but there are also many elements of danger:

- the polarization of opinion and the spreading of misinformation, often anonymously
- the transmission of hate speech and cyber-bullying, often anonymous

- the generation of anxiety and depression
- the invasion of privacy.

I will concentrate here on the last two dangers.

Platforms like Facebook and Instagram have become central to the lives of billions. They appeal to something basic in every human – the wish to be informed, to know what's going on, to be connected and to communicate. They have many advantages. But there are also some huge problems.

The first is the usual **problem of comparisons**. The more you know about other people, the more you can compare them with yourself. This is made worse by some extraordinary forms of measurement – the number of friends or followers and the number of 'Likes'.

The consequences for adolescents do seem to be quite serious. In a remarkable book, Jean Twenge has produced dozens of diagrams which tell a similar story. As the top graph in Figure 13.1 shows, time online took off from 2010 onwards, mainly due to increased use of Facebook.[22] This led to an inevitable decline in face-to-face activities. But more important were the consequences for mental health. As the lower graph shows, there was a sharp increase in the number of young people who stopped enjoying life. Also (not shown) many more of them felt 'left out' and 'lonely'.

Of course, correlation does not prove causation. But, in an ingenious randomized experiment, one group of 516 Danish adults were asked to stop using Facebook for a week, which they largely did. At the end of the week, when compared with the control group, their average life-satisfaction had increased

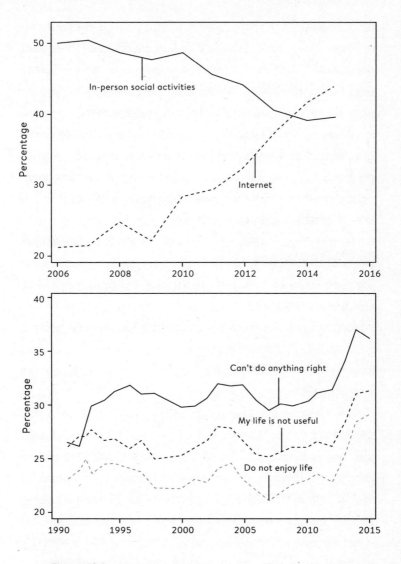

Figure 13.1
(*top*) Percentage of eighteen-year-olds spending ten or more hours per week online and percentage undertaking four face-to-face social activities
(*bottom*) Percentage of thirteen- to eighteen-year-olds experiencing negative thoughts in last twelve months

by 0.4 points (out of 10). This is a lot. Some 9 per cent fewer of them were lonely, and some 11 per cent fewer of them were depressed.[23] And in two other studies people were followed over time. After using Facebook they became less happy, and after socializing face to face they became happier.[24]

What an ironic outcome. The medium which aims to put people in touch with each other has led, instead, to more people feeling left out. Instead of living their own lives, many people have become obsessed with the lives of others – and how those lives compare with their own.

For this reason they also have to take great care **how they present themselves**. Instead of just seeing things and enjoying them, they have to post pictures of them. In many cases this is a generous deed, but in other cases it is a form of self-advertisement. Whereas earlier generations were urged not to show off, social media now invites people to do just that. The result is both anxiety for the show-off and deflation for everyone else.

Young women suffer worst because they use social media more than men. Moreover, aggression by males is typically more physical in nature and can be avoided for much of the day, while aggression by females tends to be more verbal and, if online, it's with the recipient 24/7.[25] So what is the solution? Social media will require major regulation, like most other aspects of life. All new technologies eventually get regulated. In 1930 the car (a new-fangled device) killed 7,300 people in Britain. By 2016 this number had been reduced to 1,700, largely by regulation. Regulation must be a part of the response to the internet.[26] But individuals also have to learn how to use the new technology better.[27]

A second major danger associated with social media is the **power** that it gives to those who control these platforms. This power comes from the direct access that they have to us and the knowledge they have about us. They earn their income through giving advertisers access to us and through selling data about us to banks, retailers, researchers and many others. The same is true of Google and smart phone suppliers. This use of data requires strict regulation.

One final reflection. We live in a society that is driven more and more by data. This helps us to understand the world better and to be more efficient. Science is based on data, and more and bigger data means better science. Moreover, to manage anything we need data – to know what we are achieving. We need data to manage a business and to manage a heart condition.

But, in the end, a body is more than a system of equations and so is a business. In the end, these are lived experiences. To get people to take happiness seriously, we measure it. But the measurement is only a proxy for the reality – for the subjective feeling of being alive. Measurement has an honoured place, but we are lost if it takes away the fun of life – and the magic.

Conclusions

Technology moves fast, and in 1940 no one foresaw the rise of the internet. So we can hardly guess at the technology which children born today will experience by the end of the century. But we know one thing. Basic human nature does not change. We have the same core needs as our Stone Age ancestors. We want food, shelter and physical safety. We want to be healthy and to live long. We want to love and be loved, to be respected and to be needed. We want to feel competent, independent and in control. And that's about it.

Whatever happens to technology, we will manipulate our environment to achieve these primary goals. That is what humans do. In the past we did not surrender to big business: we regulated it. In the future, we will not surrender to artificial intelligence, or to the internet giants. We will regulate them too and we will not surrender to the machine. The scientists and technologists will create the possibilities, but it is society that will decide the way we go.

Conclusion: Actions for Happiness

One candle can light a hundred other candles and continue to burn just as brightly.
— Buddha

For many people this is a good time to be alive: we are happier than people were in most previous centuries. But even in the richest countries there is still much misery. Mental illness remains common, family conflict is frequent, and work is increasingly stressful. The dominant competitive culture makes most of us unnecessarily anxious and isolated from our fellows: it is a zero-sum philosophy which cannot lead to a happier society. But a better culture is available, based on:

- one key idea
- the science of how to improve our happiness and give happiness to others, and
- the millions of people already engaged in doing just that.

The key idea

The idea comes first, because without a clear and better goal for our lives, little will change. Tinkering is not enough to solve our problems. To defeat a bad idea requires another idea that is bigger and better.

The idea is simple: that we judge our society by the happiness of the citizens, especially the happiness levels of those who are the least happy. That is the most reasonable measure of success. The goal therefore is a happier society – one where most people are happier and, above all, where fewer people are really unhappy. Some people argue against this approach, saying that there are many goods and therefore many objectives. But we cannot decide what to do unless we can compare these objectives. And, once we do that, we will find ourselves comparing them in terms of their effects on happiness – which brings us back to where we started.

So the basic principle of our **moral philosophy** should be this: that each of us tries to create the most happiness in the world that we can, especially among those who are least happy.

Many young people lack a clear purpose, and suffer from increasing problems with their mental health.[1] Here instead is an inspiring goal which puts the whole of life into perspective. It requires us to tame the egotistic side of our inherited nature and to cultivate the pro-social side. We need to develop the habit of unconditional benevolence and the capacity to feel what others feel.

The happiness goal also provides us with the basic principle of **political philosophy**: that policy-makers should try to create the most happiness they can, especially amongst those who are least happy. This, too, is an inspiring credo and can lead to much better policies, aimed especially at the relief of misery.

Science and mind-training

Ideas, however, are not enough. We also need to know how to implement them. In the last forty years there has been an explosion in the science of happiness. Research has confirmed that economic growth is no guarantee of increased happiness, especially in more advanced societies. The key factors affecting our happiness are mental health, physical health, and our human relationships – in the family, at work and in the community.

We now have new tools for improving all of these dimensions of our life. Physical health care is improving rapidly, but even more importantly we now have better ways to manage our mental life. The first breakthrough was in the treatment of mental illness. After the drug discoveries came psychological therapies like Cognitive Behavioural Therapy (CBT). These lead to recovery for over 50 per cent of people suffering from depression or from anxiety disorders like PTSD, OCD, panic attacks and social phobia. Next, the ideas behind CBT provided the basis for positive psychology, from which we can all benefit and enhance our wellbeing. At the same time, modern science has shown how different types of meditation can improve our inner calm and our capacity to empathize with others. So the greatest revolution of all can be in ourselves.

- We can achieve more control over our thoughts and feelings.
- We can develop more compassion both for others and for ourselves.

These are the tools for building a happier world.

The world happiness movement

This knowledge is already being applied by millions of people worldwide, both in their own lives and in schools, workplaces, clinics, community centres and policy-making worldwide. Figure 14.1 attempts to assemble some of the key features of the world happiness movement that we have been discussing in this book.

This movement involves millions of people who believe there is more to life than income and success, and that the ultimate reality for humans is how we feel. Most obviously, there are the users of Eastern practices (mindfulness, meditation and spiritual forms of yoga) and of Western practices (positive psychology and the different forms of self-help). Not all of them subscribe precisely to the Happiness Principle, but most of them come close to it. The same is true of most mental-health workers – one of the world's most rapidly growing professions, especially if we include counsellors and life coaches.

Then we come to the huge number of enlightened teachers, managers, community workers and volunteers, consciously trying to enhance the happiness of those around them. All of them have a similar aim – to produce not GDP but lives that flourish. Finally, we have the smaller number of enlightened policy-makers in each country and the researchers who support their efforts. The star organization here is the OECD, the club of rich nations. But wellbeing is becoming, to some extent, an objective of many governments, with inter-governmental meetings organized both by the OECD and the World Government Summit, as well as by the World Happiness Summit. Two major annual international

- **Users of meditation, mindfulness or spiritual forms of yoga**
  Some key leaders: the Dalai Lama, Jon Kabat-Zinn, Matthieu Ricard, Thich Nhat Hanh, Richard Davidson, Sharon Salzberg, Mark Williams, Jay Shetty. Some key organizations: Buddhist Societies, Art of Living Foundation, Mind & Life Institute.

- **Users of positive psychology and other forms of self-help**
  Some key leaders: Martin Seligman, Daniel Goleman, Barbara Fredrickson, Deepak Chopra, Mo Gawdat, Goldie Hawn, Oprah Winfrey, Ruby Wax, Mark Williamson.
  Some key organizations: International Positive Psychology Association, Sunday Assemblies, School of Life, Alcoholics Anonymous, Narcotics Anonymous, Action for Happiness.

- **Mental health workers, counsellors, life coaches, and their clients**
  Some key leaders: David Clark, Vikram Patel, Carolyn Webster-Stratton, Peter Fonagy, Alan Kazdin, Tal Ben-Shahar.
  Some key organizations: professional associations and associations of users.

- **Educators teaching the skills of living**
  Some key leaders: Mark Greenberg, Anthony Seldon, Angela Duckworth, Peter Singer.
  Some key organizations: International Positive Education Network, Effective Altruism, Humanist Associations.

- **Managers and others promoting happiness at work**
  Some key leaders: Arianna Huffington, Tony Hsieh, Shawn Achor.
  Some key organizations: Thrive Global, Delivering Happiness.

- **Policy experts promoting wellbeing**
  Some key leaders: Jeffrey Sachs, Gus O'Donnell, Martine Durand, Ohood al Roumi.
  Some key organizations: OECD, Sustainable Development Solutions Network, World Government Summit, World Happiness Summit (WOHASU).

- **Researchers providing the evidence-base**
  Some key leaders: Richard Easterlin, Ed Diener, Daniel Kahneman, Andrew Oswald, Andrew Clark, Bruno Frey, John Helliwell, Angus Deaton.
  Some key publications: World Happiness Report, Global Happiness and Wellbeing Policy Report, *The Origins of Happiness*.

Figure 14.1 The world happiness movement

publications support this effort: the World Happiness Report and the Global Happiness and Wellbeing Policy Report.

Who can do what?

So how can different groups contribute to a happier world? We have a mass of evidence on this. It includes some of the experiments we have discussed earlier and which are summarized in Table 14.1. And from all of this evidence there emerges clear guidance for people in different walks of life.

TEACHERS

If you want to predict whether a child will have a satisfying adult life, the most important thing is whether the child is happy, not the grades they achieve. Schools have much more effect on their children's happiness than most people think. So schools should have the happiness and values of their children as major goals. To achieve this rebalancing of priorities, schools should measure the wellbeing of the children (and its progress) on a regular basis, as they do throughout the Netherlands.

To improve wellbeing will often require a major change in the ethos of the school. In addition children can be taught to be happier and more compassionate by using evidence-based materials throughout their school life. This should become standard practice. It should not worsen exam performance, but rather improve it. And teachers should be offered courses on mental health and on classroom management, based on the evidence of what works.

MANAGERS

For most people, work is the least enjoyable experience of the day, worse even than housework. And the worst time of all is when people are with their line manager. So the philosophy of most line managers needs to change. If work is organized so that more value is placed on the happiness of the workers, this reduces the quit-rate of workers and increases both productivity and the bottom line. But, more importantly, it improves the workers' quality of life.

In order for this to happen, workers need to have more control over how their work is organized. They need a less competitive working atmosphere, with an end to 'forced ranking' of team members. Managers need to be selected for their ability to inspire as well as to organize, and they need courses on how to do that. They also need to understand mental illness and to get help for their workers if they are struggling. And, of course, firms should measure worker wellbeing and print the results on the front page of their Annual Report.

HEALTH WORKERS

We need a revolution in health care. Someone who is suffering from mental-health problems should be as likely to get the best available treatment as someone with a physical illness. That is what parity of esteem for mental health means. The treatment should have good evidence of success, which means proper measurement of its outcome. Good treatments averaging under ten sessions now exist for depression and anxiety disorders, but even in the richest countries most people who need them do not get them. Such treatments pay

Intervention	Impact
By schools	
Good Behaviour Game (at age 6)	Anti-social behaviour halved (at age 20)
Healthy Minds (140 hours from age 11–15)	Life-satisfaction increased by 7% points (at age 15)
Positive Education (100 hours, secondary school)	Wellbeing and academic performance up by 8–19% points (one year later)
By managers	
STAR participatory programme (8 hours for team, 12 hours for manager)	Job satisfaction up 11% points and quitting down by 1/3 (after 6 months)
Working from home (call centres)	Life-satisfaction +18%; productivity +13%; quitting −50% (after 9 months)
Stopping forced ranking (of sales reps)	Sales +11%
By health workers	
CBT for anxiety/depression (average 7 sessions)	Recovery during treatment 50%, depression relapse halved
Anti-depressants (for severe depression)	Recovery during treatment 50%, relapse unaffected unless drugs continue
Incredible Years (10 group sessions for parents of disturbed young children)	Conduct disorder −80% (10 years later)
CBT for couples in conflict (10 sessions)	50% of couples now satisfied with the relationship (after 6 months)

Intervention	Impact
By communities	
Experience Corps (over 60s giving literacy support to children)	Growth of hippocampal and cortical brain areas (after 2 years)
Loneliness prevention (old people in day-care centres)	Subjective health +25%
By individuals	
Exploring What Matters	Life-satisfaction up 20% points

Table 14.1
Some effective interventions

for themselves through the amount they save on welfare benefits and extra physical health care.

So in every country much more needs to be spent on mental health. Of course, physical health is also a major factor affecting happiness (and length of life). So, as countries get richer, the share of GDP going on health care, both physical and mental, has to rise. And the use of narcotic drugs should be treated as a health problem, not an issue of criminal justice.

FAMILIES

Family relationships are crucial to our happiness. If conflict occurs within the family, there are excellent treatments of around ten sessions, which can frequently restore lost love, even after domestic violence or infidelity. However, it would be better to prevent these conflicts from arising in the first place, often after the first child arrives. So all parents should be offered ante-natal classes which cover not only physical childbirth and childcare, but the relationship between the parents and their relationship with the child. And, if the child develops behavioural problems, there are excellent training courses for parents in how to help their child. Once the child is over one year old, there is no reason why both parents should not work. But at that point there has to be good childcare available, and at the time of childbirth there must be generous parental leave.

COMMUNITIES

Everybody needs to feel they belong. They need to belong to a family, to belong at work, and to belong to a local community. Some communities feel more friendly than others, with individuals genuinely engaging with each other. Happy communities are characterized by high levels of volunteering, a physical layout which encourages a sense of belonging, and typically an adequate amount of green space. But two factors can undermine the feeling of belonging: crime and ethnic differences. The solution to these is not to retreat into the bunker; it is to endeavour skilfully to reach out to the ex-prisoner and the migrant, and draw them into the community.

ECONOMISTS

Economists are different from any of the groups we have considered so far. They have two roles. One is to introduce a revolution in policy-making, where all policies get judged by how they contribute to the happiness of the people. The second role is to press for better management of the economy itself. In that sphere priority should go, not to long-term growth, but to economic stability. There should be a low level of unemployment, secured by an active labour market policy and a guarantee of work after one year of unemployment. Income inequality should be reduced by ensuring that everyone gets a decent level of skill. Wherever possible, we should help people to earn a decent life for themselves, rather than hand them cash. And poor countries should not go for helter-skelter growth, but for a pattern of development that maintains or creates meaningful communities. Uncontrolled international migration cannot be the answer to world poverty, since it would lead to unmanageable tensions.

SCIENTISTS AND TECHNOLOGISTS

Ultimately, the material basis of our society will be decided by the scientists and engineers. Pure science must be driven by pure curiosity. But for applied research priority should surely be given to those inventions which are most likely to increase human happiness.

First among these should be cheap, clean energy. The only sure way to protect our climate is to make clean energy cheaper to produce than dirty energy. Until recently only 4 per cent of publicly funded research in the world has been on the production of clean energy. Mission Innovation is doubling that, and hopefully clean energy research will attract the brightest and best of our young scientists.

Second come discoveries that will reduce pain, especially mental pain. At present under 5 per cent of medical research goes on mental health. Third, I would suggest, come robots. Billions of people do work which is either back-breaking or boring. Robots can replace these jobs, releasing those displaced to do more interesting work – provided they are given the necessary skills.

As a social scientist, I should end with social science. It is the job of social scientists to discover the causes of happiness and misery – direct and indirect. It is also their job to organize thousands of detailed experiments to find out how we can best promote the happiness of our people.

POLITICIANS

But in the end it is the politicians who will make the key decisions. Their goal should be the happiness of the people – the new ideology should be the Happiness Principle. This should

- Our single purpose is to help people live happier lives.

- We will revolutionize the treatment of mental illness and addiction and ensure that people with mental-health problems have the same access to state-of-the-art treatment as people with physical health problems.

- We will transform the goals of education to include the wellbeing of students, measuring it and giving it the same priority as their academic learning.

- We will support families not only financially where necessary, but also by offering training in the arts of parenting, help with difficult children, and support with family conflict and domestic violence.

- We will ensure that all young people are welcomed into the world of work and given the skills they need to be fruitfully employed.

- Our macro-economic policies will give priority to economic stability over faster long-term growth.

- As employers, we will give high priority to the morale and job satisfaction of public sector workers.

- We will develop every community so that it provides a sense of belonging and opportunities for social connection and voluntary activity to every citizen.

- We will combat climate change for the sake of our children and grandchildren, with the use of science and financial incentives to restrain and then halt the growth of greenhouse gases.

- We will decriminalize the use of narcotic drugs and treat it as a problem of health and not of criminal justice.

- We will build a more egalitarian ethos which replaces the appeal to greed by an appeal to the common good.

- And, in all we do, we will use evidence to husband our resources and spend money only on those policies which contribute most to the happiness of the people.

Figure 14.2
The election manifesto of a party focused on people's wellbeing

be the goal of every government and it should be the guiding principle behind each party's political manifesto. So what difference would it make if politics was about the happiness of the people? What would be the new priorities? Here is my first draft of an election manifesto for a party focused on people's wellbeing (see Figure 14.2).

Each of us

That is the view from the top down. But in the end what matters even more is what comes from the bottom up. I have left until last the role of each of us as individuals. In the end, it is our goals that will determine the happiness of our society. The goal of personal success is a dead end since it is zero-sum; it will not produce the greater happiness we desire. Instead, we need a positive-sum culture which focuses explicitly on creating a happier world.

We need individuals who consciously commit themselves to creating as much happiness as they can for others and for themselves. These aims are not generally in conflict. Helping others is the surest way to avoid self-absorption, but we do also need to care for our own happiness and to develop a technique for being happy whatever happens to us. Such techniques may not always work. But as Abraham Lincoln (who was a depressive) once said, 'Most folks are as happy as they make up their minds to be.' We owe it to ourselves to manage our emotions and to find things to celebrate day by day.

To live well is not easy. It is much easier if you meet regularly with others of like mind, to be supported, comforted and inspired. This has been one role for the churches, mosques, synagogues and temples throughout the ages. But we live in an increasingly secular age and now we need a secular ethic. We also need secular organizations that embody that spirit. That is why Action for Happiness was founded, with the Dalai Lama as patron. It now has 130,000 members in 180 countries, and over a million followers online. It has groups that meet regularly after taking the eight-session course on Exploring What Matters, and it is growing rapidly.

So whether you belong to an organization like Action for Happiness or to none, I wonder whether you would like to consider what you will do differently in your life as a result of reading this book. It's up to you, but if you would like to, feel free to record whatever new ideas you have about how you might make the world a better place.

MY PERSONAL MANIFESTO TO MYSELF

Conclusion

The world happiness movement is a house of many rooms. It is not a movement of drop-outs; it is a movement of people who want to engage passionately in the welfare of others, while taking care of their own inner space.

There is no objective reason why so many lives in the West should be so stressful. We ourselves have created the stress by our goals, and the way our institutions respond to them. If we change our goals, we really can produce a happier society.

Future generations will be shocked by many of the unthinking and unskilful features of life today. They will be shocked at the neglect of mental illness, at the stresses imposed on our children, and at the common assumption that everyone is an egotist.

But cultures can be changed and change is often rapid. Until recently, men dominated the world of work, gay couples had to hide in shame, and it was fashionable to smoke in public places. Even more recently, domestic violence, child abuse and sexual harassment were swept under the carpet. But no longer. In every case it is a powerful social movement that has brought about the change.

So the world happiness movement can indeed bring in a better, gentler culture and do it fast. But what happens will ultimately depend on each one of us. We can all be heroes in the happiness revolution.

A Note of Thanks

Positive psychology encourages the writing of gratitude letters. This one will be quite long, because I would like to thank all those who have contributed most to my philosophy of life – and to say what I have learned from them. There are two things they all have in common: a generous spirit and a strong desire to improve the quality of human life.

My parents

I should begin with the German doctor who saved my father's life (and thus mine). In mental torment in Berlin, my father put a pistol in his mouth, pointing upwards. The bullet missed his brain but lodged in his skull. Following the operation to remove it, he recovered swiftly and soon met my mother. In due course I appeared. I was a love-child.

My father's basic belief was in original virtue. Children, he thought, were born happy, but were made miserable by the way they were treated. We now know more than he did about the role of genes. But it was not a bad starting point, and it was got through hard experience. After an unhappy time at Bedales School and Cambridge, he went as a barely trained anthropologist to the New Hebrides (now Vanuatu). It was the best year of his life. But he contracted malaria and spent the next ten years in a state of physical and mental break-down. He had many psychoanalysts and in the end become a leading Jungian analyst himself as well as a writer. Patients felt he was on their side and he helped many of them. But he could never relate to his equals as well as he did to his patients, and quarrelled with almost everyone except me, because I refused to quarrel with him. I experienced him as a lovely and creative father until I was ten, when he essentially left the family.

My mother by contrast was someone everyone loved. She was very positive, with a good common-sense philosophy of life. She too became a Jungian psychoanalyst, of a very practical kind. Like my father she grew up as an atheist, but in 1942 they both became Catholics – because of the symbolism and without any belief in the creed.

I was born five years before the Second World War. I was a happy child and I was brought up in a progressive way with reasons given, and I went to a progressive day school in London. But, after war broke out, we moved for safety to Oxford. There I made a wonderful friend, Peter Westwood, with whom I played every non-school day for seven years. He had as sweet a nature as any I have ever known, and most of what I know about friendship must have been learned from him. We were wartime children, but untouched by the war until the Allies started winning when I was eight years old. In Peter's garden there was an earthen air-raid shelter, rather like a long barrow. We called it the rock of Gibraltar and on it we installed gun emplacements and a hospital. One day, I'm told, a grand Oxford lady called Mrs Haldane came to look at it and saw three soldiers lying on their backs in the hospital. She said, 'Oh dear they must be feeling awful,' to which I replied, 'Not really, they're only suffering from venereal disease.'

School and Army

I went as a day-boy to the Dragon School in Oxford. This remarkable institution was not a progressive school, but it had a winning level of informality: the teachers all had nicknames. One, in particular, known as Jacko, gave me a lasting love of history. The morning assembly was focused on values, not the creed. We learned great phrases such as 'Others before self' and 'Fight the good fight with all thy might'. And of course we played team games which embodied the idea of collective effort.

At the age of thirteen the top students from the Dragon School won scholarships to Eton College or Winchester College. I went to Eton, which I loved. But the whole experience was fraught with contradiction. On the one side, it was hugely competitive. Each term there were exams which generated the 'form order' for the next term. This 'form order' determined where you sat in chapel and in lessons, and which table you sat at for your meals. On the other hand, you had to be a team player and to be modest. I was not comfortable when a winner of the Victoria Cross told us we should walk with our heads held high.

On the whole we managed the combination of competition and team spirit quite well. Academically I was in competition for top place with my dearest friend, Kit Welchman. But it didn't interfere with our friendship, and from him I learned so much about poetry and the arts. We lived in a house called College which housed all the boys who had won scholarships. It was a precocious place and we were discussing the main issues of philosophy by the age of fifteen. We were all left-wing. This was natural under the great Labour government of 1945–51, but Eton scholars at other times have often been non-conformist – including Maynard Keynes and George Orwell. When we were there, the great headmaster Robert Birley was a known Labour supporter. I already knew about the Webbs and the Fabians through my mother and, when I discussed with Kit what we wanted to do in life, I said I wanted to be a social reformer.

For me, a key aspect of school was chapel and evening prayers. We worshipped twice a day, except Sundays when it was four times. None of us believed in the afterlife, miracles, the virgin birth, the resurrection or the ascension. But we believed in God, transcendent and imminent; in trying to fulfil our appointed roles; and in accepting whatever happened to us. On the war memorial were inscribed the words from Milton's 'Samson Agonistes':

> All is best, though we oft doubt,
> What th' unsearchable dispose
> Of highest wisdom brings about,
> And ever best found in the close.

And we had a strong belief in 'calm of mind, all passion spent'. We believed that one should cultivate noble feelings, and, when my father came to tell me that he and Mum were getting divorced, I duly reacted 'more in sorrow than in anger'. We evaluated the masters and older boys according to whether they were 'great men', noble in spirit. One master, Brian

Young, we admired particularly. He taught us about Aristotle and the great-hearted person. We deplored pomposity, but loved the concept of the happy mean. This included the idea that life should involve a lot more than work – friendship, poetry, acting, painting, music (clarinet) and of course sport. In the sixth form I specialized first in classics. But one day an egregious preacher stated that 'before Jesus, no one smiled'. I thought I had better study history.

After school, we all went into the Army. I chose the Artillery, a non-Etonian regiment, and was stationed in Germany as an officer at Belsen, renamed Hohne. I enjoyed it a lot – the technical aspects of gunnery, but above all working with men from every kind of background. In my first week I drove my 3-tonne lorry into a cul-de-sac in a forest. At that moment my battery commander Marcus Lipton arrived. I was mortified, and even more alarmed on the next day when he sent for me. But, instead of mentioning my failings, he gave me additional responsibility. I have never forgotten that lesson on trust.

Cambridge

Next came King's College, Cambridge, where I took a degree in history. From reading Jeremy Bentham and John Stuart Mill I quickly became a utilitarian (though modified by a preference for equality of happiness). King's was a stimulating environment, more encouraging of non-conformity than Eton, and I learned more from student societies and fellow students than from the teachers. From my second term I belonged to the Apostles, a small group that had met every week for earnest debate since 1830 and had included Tennyson, Keynes and Bertrand Russell. This was a major influence on me and through it I duly lost my Christian faith.

That process accelerated when the Dean of the college threw himself from the roof of the great chapel on to the hard paving stones below. From then on I rapidly became a humanist (but with a touch of pantheism). I also concluded that mental health was a major issue, as my father had already taught me. So I asked the tutor of the college, John Raven, whether I could study psychiatry. The college generously agreed to finance this. I had to take four A level exams in physics, chemistry, biology and organic chemistry, which I did in a year, and then moved on to dissect head and neck, and thorax. By then I was twenty-five. Medical students were treated with less respect than history students and I realized I couldn't continue being a student. But I am extremely grateful that I learned the science which has stood me in good stead in my studies of happiness.

Instead of pursuing medicine I became a history teacher in a comprehensive school. This was a lovely experience, putting me in touch with an even wider range of people than the army. It filled me with belief in the educability of nearly everybody. I expected to remain in teaching and teacher-training for the rest of my life. However, in the evenings I was going to the London School of Economics (LSE) to broaden my mind with a course on sociology. As part of that I had taken a class with the statistician Claus Moser, who was to change my life.

The Robbins Committee

Claus was appointed adviser to the so-called Robbins Committee on Higher Education and asked me to become its senior research officer. It was an extraordinary experience – a real voyage of discovery. It had not occurred to me (or to most of my generation) that one could study the present in a scientific way. For the Robbins Committee I organized three big surveys and wrote four appendix volumes, as well as short sections of the report. Most importantly we demolished the idea of the so-called 'pool of ability' which opened the way to mass higher education in Britain. Philosophically, I learned for the first time about the wonderful concept of cost–benefit analysis, which could be applied to anything including educational policy. So, when the writing of the report was ending and I was asked to work on educational policy at the London School of Economics (LSE), I readily agreed.

Economics

But my first week at the LSE revealed an awful truth. I could not do this job without becoming an economist. So I had to become a student again at the age of thirty-one. What a change. Until then I had been someone born with a silver spoon in his mouth, for whom most things came easily. Now I was ten years behind. For years it was a real struggle, but in the end I was rescued by a sequence of wonderful colleagues, who further extended my intellectual horizons.

The first of these was Amartya Sen. When I joined the economics department at the LSE it was mostly very right-wing – and not too different from Milton Friedman's department at Chicago. I felt uncomfortable questioning the free market orthodoxy. And then Amartya arrived. He treated me with respect and we ran a seminar on Equality together – it generated massive interest. From Amartya I also learned a huge amount about the theory of social choice and the conditions necessary for the Happiness Principle to be valid. Though he has become less enthusiastic about the principle, we are not far apart when one considers the whole spectrum of objectives that different people support, from GDP at one end to happiness at the other.

Another surprising supporter was Alan Walters. Though very right-wing and later an adviser to Margaret Thatcher, he was a strong meritocrat with many left-wing friends. For many years I taught the microeconomics course that Alan started, and eventually turned it into what Amartya called the most left-wing microeconomics textbook around. It was Alan more than anyone who taught me that, if you want to influence policy, you should get to know politicians.

But the two economists to whom I owe the most are Richard Jackman and Stephen Nickell. In 1974 the LSE formed the Centre for Labour Economics, with me as Director. It later evolved into the Centre for Economic Performance (CEP), superbly administered by Nigel Rogers. Initially we worked on inequality, but in 1979 unemployment rose to new heights. So, for ten years in the 1980s, we ran a weekly seminar and an annual international conference to get to the bottom of what was going on. Richard is wonderfully intuitive and insistent on rigour. Steve is not only that, but also a powerful mathematician and an indefatigable collector of relevant evidence – one of the best economists of his generation. Both have massive common sense, and working with them on unemployment has been one of the best experiences of my life.

After 1979 unemployment in the UK remained high for many years. It did not feel enough to write about it; we wanted to influence the British government. For some years I had known the delightful politician Shirley Williams and through her I helped the new Social Democratic Party to develop a coherent set of labour market policies. But in 1984 we decided to launch a cross-party movement to reduce unemployment, by reforming the way unemployed people were treated (on the supply side) together with demand expansion. We founded the Employment Institute and my wife Molly ran a parallel Campaign for Work. These organizations had a significant influence on the Conservative government, but more on the Labour opposition, which at the time had an employment spokesman called Tony Blair. In due course Tony Blair and Gordon Brown implemented many of our proposals, and persuaded European leaders like Gerhard Schroeder to follow suit.

All these efforts were helped greatly by our economist colleagues based in the United States. The first of these was the outstanding labour economist Orley Ashenfelter, who has been a huge supporter of our work over the years. But then something unusual happened. I was invited to join a five-person European Macroeconomic Policy Group chaired by Rudi Dornbusch. Rudi was not only a brilliant macroeconomist but hugely inspirational – he made you feel you could do things you never dreamed of. We met regularly in Brussels and later regrouped as the WIDER World Economy

Group. The other key member of the group was Olivier Blanchard, a macroeconomist who is equally at home in labour economics and in macro. Many of our ideas about unemployment emerged somewhere in the space between Olivier and ourselves. Olivier and I later visited Poland three times as it emerged from Communism, and he has remained a friend and supporter to this day. Finally, I must mention Stanley Fischer. We have never worked together, but Stan has been a huge support and a wonderful friend. On one occasion I called him when he was No. 2 at the IMF and he asked me to lunch the next day, at which point he produced the *New Yorker* cartoon with which I began my book, *Happiness*. All three of these friends (Rudi, Olivier and Stan) have been strong supporters of my work on happiness. And it was Rudi who got me involved in Russia.

Russia

Our big book on unemployment was published in 1991 and in the same year Russia rejected Communism. Earlier that year I had visited the institute run by Yegor Gaidar and we had planned a joint research project to begin in August 1991. In the week before going to Moscow, my wife and I were holidaying in Yalta. One day we learned that Gorbachev had been imprisoned nearby by a group of reactionaries. However, within days this counter-revolution had collapsed and Gorbachev was released, but discredited. Boris Yeltsin came to power and the following November invited Gaidar to form a government. Gaidar asked me to be an adviser to one of the other Deputy Prime Ministers, and I was given an office on the floor beneath Stalin's old office. However, it was not easy working at that level – things moved so fast and they happened in Russian. Again I was very lucky. I moved one level down to work with Sergei Vasiliev, a brilliant and well-placed official in Gaidar's group. We worked together for five years. Our team produced *Russian Economic Trends* each month, which included an up-to-date analysis of the whole economy, plus an in-depth analysis of one new topic. The report was presented by me at a Russian government official press conference each month, chaired by Sergei. From my time in Russia I learned the importance of culture in human history.

Apprenticeship

In 1997 Labour came to power in Britain and in 2000 I was made a Labour member of the House of Lords. I had been advising the Labour Party on labour market policy since 1990, and from 1997 to 2001 I was a part-time consultant to David Blunkett, the remarkable Secretary of State for Education and Employment, and his Minister of State, Tessa Blackstone, a lifelong friend and supporter. It was a great chance to help implement ideas I had been developing for years. The first of these was active help to unemployed people in return for the ending of life on benefits. The second was the development of a proper system of apprenticeship. For years Hilary Steedman and I had been advocating a system in which the main alternative to university was apprenticeship – learning while earning. Apprenticeship had in earlier times been the main route to social mobility, and we argued that it should become as automatically available to less academic children as the academic route was to those who were suited to it. It took a decade to convert the Labour leadership to this view, and in

2009 they passed the Apprenticeships, Skills, Children and Learning Act which guaranteed an apprenticeship to anyone qualified. Two years later the Conservatives repealed this clause. But by then apprenticeship had established itself as a fashionable concept in Britain, even if subject to constant changes of policy.

Happiness

During the 1990s I became increasingly aware of the progress of happiness research. Among economists in Britain, this was led by Andrew Oswald, first from within our Centre for Economic Research (CEP) and then at Warwick University. But a key figure in the field was the psychologist Daniel Kahneman, who later won the Nobel Prize for economics. We invited him to give three public lectures at the LSE in 1998. He told me of the neuro-scientific research of Richard Davidson which shows that the subjective experience of happiness is an objective electro-chemical phenomenon that is measured reasonably well by what people say. So in early 2001 I decided it was time to remake the case for the Happiness Principle, since we now had the science to make it a practical proposition. That has remained my main purpose ever since – to get individuals and policy-makers to use our knowledge to create a happier world.

Improving access to psychological therapy

The book I wrote on *Happiness* (2005) clearly struck a chord and was translated into nineteen other languages. But I wanted to apply it in practice, so I asked Ed Miliband if I could write a paper on mental health for Gordon Brown.

Instead it became a paper for the No. 10 Policy Unit. It was written with help from my wife and presented at a Cabinet Office seminar in January 2005. The key figure at that seminar was David Clark. One of the world's leading clinical psychologists, David is also an incredible persuader and organizer, who since then has devoted his life to creating the Improving Access to Psychological Therapy (IAPT) service. This was launched in 2008, but it was not a foregone conclusion. There was an election commitment to the idea, but then massive resistance. The idea was said to be 'unevidenced and too expensive'. It took sixty one-on-one meetings to persuade everyone who needed to be persuaded. I later discovered that at key meetings it took only one person to say the idea was controversial for it to be blocked. But, thanks to support from the Prime Minister, Gordon Brown, it was eventually funded. However, even after that, the programme was threatened with collapse in 2012 when the job of improving health care was handed over from the Department of Health to the newly created board of the National Health Service. The NHS decided to continue all the six physical health-care development programmes (e.g. on cancer and heart disease), but it judged the IAPT development programme was now mature enough to be dropped. I still have the letter. In fact the service was only 25 per cent of the way to maturity and without further national leadership it would have deteriorated rapidly. That was when being a member of the House of Lords helped. I let the NHS know that if they did not change their minds, I would make a dreadful row in Parliament. Eventually, the NHS relented and the service has gone from strength to strength.

Child mental health

The key challenge now is to secure a deal for children with mental health problems – something similar to what we have for adults. Our basic proposal was developed jointly with the child psychiatrist Stephen Scott when I was drafting the Good Childhood Report, published in 2009. Ten years later it has now been accepted, but implementation is only just beginning.

Of course prevention is even better than cure. A key figure here is Martin Seligman, a leading psychologist and founder of positive psychology. I had learned much from him and in 2007 a CEP-led consortium did a trial of his Penn Resilience Programme in twenty schools. In it, eleven-year-olds received eighteen hours of special instruction. The programme was moderately successful, but I concluded that if we wished to transform children's lives we should spend more than eighteen hours in doing so. So we formed the Healthy Minds consortium to trial a programme lasting an hour a week over four years. It has been very well organized (by Lucy Bailey) and well taught (by Emma Judge) and the results are discussed in Chapter 6.

Happiness and public policy

These are useful achievements, but what we really want is for all public policy to be directed at the goal of happiness. The key figure here has been Gus O'Donnell, who was a brilliant head of the UK Treasury and then its top civil servant and Cabinet Secretary. A long-time believer in the happiness objective, he made major efforts to move policy in that direction. With the backing of the prime minister, David Cameron, he introduced the annual measurement of national subjective wellbeing and made it an official national statistic. Since leaving the civil service he has worked tirelessly to make the Happiness Principle the goal of government. In 2014 he chaired a committee on what this would involve – and the resulting report is still the definitive work on this topic.[1] And in 2014 he got the government to establish a What Works Centre for Wellbeing which aims to collect the research evidence into a form where it can be used by British policy-makers. Our small research group at the CEP has formed part of that Centre.

Some years back it became clear that policy-makers could not evaluate policy in terms of its impact on happiness without a large, organized, research base. They needed to know how every conceivable experience affected a person's happiness – in quantitative terms. This required original research on a range of datasets, but always using the same method of analysis. We carried this out with the help of an excellent team at the LSE and it was published in 2018 as *The Origins of Happiness* (by Andrew Clark et al.). With Gus and others I'm continuing to press the case for happiness-based policies in Britain – using, among other things, a dining club where we interact with key ministers and policy-makers.

In the meantime, there have been major developments on the international front. A key figure has been the leading economist Jeffrey Sachs. Once a strong free-marketeer, he has become one of the strongest challengers of neoconservatism and a passionate believer in the happiness objective. In conjunction with the former Prime Minister of

Bhutan, he organized a conference on happiness in 2011. It was during that conference that he invented the idea of the annual World Happiness Report, edited by him, John Helliwell and myself. John Helliwell is an amazingly resourceful economist and his analyses of the Gallup World Poll have enlarged our understanding of the causes of happiness, but also generated interest in the subject in every single country.

Action for Happiness

However, in the end, it is the citizens of the world who will decide the direction of our culture. That is why Anthony Seldon, Geoff Mulgan and I decided to form Action for Happiness. Geoff had been head of policy for Tony Blair and had tried unsuccessfully to interest him in the happiness objective. Anthony had boldly introduced the teaching of happiness into the curriculum at Wellington College, the secondary school where he was head. We were unbelievably fortunate to find Mark Williamson, who became the full-time director of the movement. With few resources Mark has worked wonders, and the public's reaction confirms that there is a huge demand for such an organization. It is my dearest wish that it can provide the spiritual and moral uplift for which people are looking worldwide.

On this score I need to mention one other thing. In 1995 my wife and I began attending the Hampstead Quaker Meeting. This rekindled my interest in the inner life. We belonged to a small Quaker study group and met every month for five years with two other couples (the Barneses and the Gilberts) from whom we learned so much. This experience inspired my belief that there is a huge role for regular meetings that can inspire and uplift people in a secular age. And that is what Action for Happiness aims to provide.

As for my own beliefs, I was asked recently by my LSE colleague Tim Besley what I believed. I attach my answer as online Annex 15.1.

Conclusion

So if you ask me where my attitudes and ideas come from, I would have to say, 'All of the above'. From my parents I got the progressive viewpoint that each person is a child of circumstance and we should empathize with everyone. From Eton I got the idea of acceptance and the desire to make a difference, while Cambridge introduced me to secular ethics.

But it was economics which gave me, for the first time, a way to think about public policy, and it also made me look at the quantitative aspect, which is essential for public policy. At one point I wrote a book about traditional cost–benefit analysis. But without the pioneering work of Ed Diener and Andrew Oswald I would never have dreamed that economics could be expanded to tackle the huge range of human problems for which traditional cost–benefit analysis is inadequate.

And the same applies to the issue of cultural change and secular ethics. I never liked the ultra-competitive culture spreading out of the USA. But how to tackle the selfish side of our nature? From the Quakers, from CBT and from the Dalai Lama I learned that we can all gain some control over our inner life and increase our compassion for ourselves and for others. But to create an organization to push these ideas required the chutzpah supplied by the other co-founders of Action for

Happiness. The happiness movement in all its forms is going well and I'm confident that history is on our side – both in the public policy arena and in the hearts of people.

Though I have done a number of different things since 1964, I have always been at the London School of Economics. I have worked there for fifty-six years. It has been a uniformly happy experience. The LSE is an amazing institution, where people really help each other and where you can pursue almost any interest that you believe to be important. Within the LSE, the Centre for Economic Performance – where I still work – has always been a happy place and it continues to go from strength to strength. In my years at the LSE I have had only four assistants: Pam Mounsey, Marion O'Brien, Harriet Ogborn and Jo Cantlay. They have all been wonderful, and without them I could have done nothing.

This book

On this book, the hero is George Ward. He is one of the two brightest young researchers I have ever known and a virtual co-author of the book. We planned every chapter together; he researched the literature, did further analysis and greatly improved the resulting chapters. Another hero is Jo Cantlay, who handled the many drafts of the manuscript so brilliantly, from beginning to end. Friends and colleagues have been extremely generous with the time they have given to commenting on the book. In September 2018 David Clark kindly hosted a two-day conference on the draft of the book at his beautiful Magdalen College in Oxford. Those who came were Tim Besley, Jan De Neve, John Helliwell, David King, Paul Litchfield, Molly Meacher, Gus O'Donnell, Michael Plant, Anthony Seldon,

Peter Singer (online) and Mark Williamson. They all made huge contributions and have massively improved the book. I have also had great help from Oriana Bandiera, Don Baucom, Andrew Clark, John Collins, Carolyn Cowan, Paul Frijters, David Halpern, Gordon Harrold, Vanessa King, Christian Krekel, Sonia Livingstone, Geoff Mulgan, Stephen Scott and Richard Wilkinson. As with earlier books, I have been incredibly lucky to have such a wonderful agent in Caroline Dawnay and such an outstanding Penguin editor as Stuart Proffitt, who much improved the draft. I am so grateful for all their support.

In my private life I have also been blessed, though it took me until I was fifty-one to find my ideal woman. Molly is brilliant, caring and lovely. She goes straight to the heart of every issue; she campaigns fearlessly; and I love her look. From the beginning she has been a huge supporter of my work on happiness – and on mental health, which she knows more about than I do. This book would not have been written without her. And she has brought me four wonderful step-children (David, Nigel, Sally and Ros), nine amazing grandchildren (Tom, Maddy, Lovis, Elizabeth, Mark, Lucy, Lauren, Dylan and Violet) – and our lovely tennis group. What more could I want?

Thank you all so much.

Richard

Sources of Figures and Tables

Figure 0.2 (*top*) Articles in *The Guardian* newspaper mentioning happiness and mental health
Factiva Global News Database.

Figure 0.2 (*bottom left*) Articles on happiness in academic journals
Taken from the number of papers in the EconLit and Web of Science databases with reference in the title or abstract to: subjective wellbeing, subjective well-being, life-satisfaction, happy, or happiness.

Figure 0.2 (*bottom right*) Google searches for meditation and yoga
Google Trends. Figures refer to searches in the USA. All figures are normalized on the total number of searches in a given period. For each series, Jan 2008 = 100.

Figure 1.3 How occupations differ in average happiness and average salary in the UK
O'Donnell et al. (2014), p. 72. Numbers relate to mid-career life-satisfaction.

Figure 1.4 Average happiness of British people in each decile of happiness
Gallup World Poll (Answers to the 'Cantril Ladder' question: *Please imagine a ladder with steps numbered from 0 at the bottom to 10 at the top. Suppose we say that the top of the ladder represents the best possible life for you and the bottom of the ladder represents the worst possible life for you. If the top step is*

*10 and the bottom step is 0, on which step of the ladder do you
feel you personally stand at the present time?*). Average = 6.7:
Standard deviation = 1.87 for 2015–2017.

Figure 2.1 Happiness affects longevity
Data supplied by Andrew Steptoe. See also Steptoe and
Wardle (2012).

Figure 2.2 What explains the variation of adult happiness
(in Britain)?
A. E. Clark et al. (2018), Table 16.1. For quality of work index,
see p. 74 of that book and chapter 7 of this book. The β-
coefficient is 0.20 for the employed population, but for all
adults it becomes 0.16 (0.20 times the square root of the
employment rate).

Table 2.1 Ranking of countries by their average happiness (on the
scale 0–10)
Gallup World Poll. Years 2016–2018. Replies based on the
Cantril ladder.

Table 2.2 How is national happiness (0–10) affected by national
variables?
Private information from John Helliwell and Haifang Huang.
Closely related to Helliwell, Layard and Sachs (2018), Table 2.1,
column 1, but including trust and excluding corruption. These
trust data are available for one year only and cover 128 countries.

Figure 2.3 Stress is increasing
Gallup World Poll.

Figure 4.1 US students have become more materialistic
Twenge (2017), Figure 6.8, p. 168 (American Freshman Survey
1967–2016).

Figure 4.2. A Norwegian newspaper reflects increasing
individualism and reduced communal values
Nafstad et al. (2007)

Figure 5.1 Percentage saying that they had a great deal of confidence in the church or organized religion (USA)
Gallup (http://www.gallup.com/poll/1690/religion.aspx)

Figure 5.2 Ten Keys to Happier Living
Action for Happiness website.

Figure 5.3 The Exploring What Matters course has big effects (two months later)
Krekel et al. (2020).

Figure 6.1 (*top*) What predicts happiness at age sixteen?
A. E. Clark et al. (2018), Figure 1.5(b).

Figure 6.1 (*bottom*) What in childhood predicts a happy adult?
A. E. Clark et al. (2018), Figure 1.2.

Table 6.1 Fewer children feel comfortable in school (OECD)
OECD (2017), Fig. III.7.1, p. 119. OECD average of thirty countries, including all OECD countries, with the exception of Chile, Estonia, Israel, Slovenia and the United States. All changes are statistically significant.

Figure 6.2 Wellbeing teaching improves wellbeing and academic performance (Bhutan)
Adler (2016). See also Seligman and Adler (2018). Results after completing a fifteen-month course of two hours per week. One year later these gains remain largely unchanged.

Figure 7.1 Unhappiness depends on who you are with (USA)
Krueger (2009), Table 1.10. US Adults. This shows how much of the time the dominant emotion is unpleasant.

Figure 7.2 Unhappiness depends on what you are doing
Krueger (2009), Table 1.9.

Figure 7.3 How job satisfaction is affected by different aspects of workplace organization
De Neve (2018), cross-section, ISSP.

Figure 7.4 How the STAR experiment improved wellbeing at work
   Moen et al. (2016). We focus on results for the experiment
   before the company was merged with another company. Effect
   sizes are taken from Table 2, Panel A. Standardized effect sizes
   are calculated using the usual-practice control group standard
   deviations of each measure.

Figure 8.1 How much misery is explained by each factor?
   A. E. Clark et al. (2018), Table 6.2, p. 94. Note: These are
   partial correlation coefficients explaining misery (taken as a 0/1
   variable). Income is entered negatively as a continuous variable.

Figure 8.2 Mental illness makes death more likely
   E. Walker et al. (2015). These are annual death rates, adjusted
   for age and gender. Global analysis.

Figure 8.3 Foreign aid discriminates against mental illness
   Gilbert et al. (2015) and Charlson et al. (2017).

Figure 8.4 Age at which people died in the UK – 1910
   compared to 2016
   Human Mortality Database, Period Life Table for England
   and Wales. Deaths at age 0 not plotted (1910: 10.6 per cent;
   2016: 0.4 per cent).

Table 10.1 Percentage of people who feel lonely in Britain
   Thomas (2015). Percentage answering 6 or above.

Figure 11.1 Unemployment in Western Europe
   OECD.Stat database. The years 2015 and earlier show the
   percentage of the civilian labour force; the years 2016–2017
   show the percentage of the total labour force.

Table 11.1 Inequality has risen in some English-speaking countries
   and less elsewhere
   Gross weekly earnings. OECD.Stat database. (Full-time male
   employees)

Table 11.2 Average cost of reducing the numbers in misery, by one person
A. E. Clark et al. (2016). For methods of calculation, see online Annex 11.1.

Figure 11.2 Average happiness in China, using five studies, 1990–2015
Helliwell, Layard and Sachs (2017), Figure 3.1. WVS is World Values Survey and CGSS is Chinese General Social Survey.

Figure 12.1 Factors explaining the vote share of the existing government parties (European elections, 1970–2014)
Ward (forthcoming).

Figure 12.2 Conduct of government and average happiness
Gallup World Poll; World Bank. Average happiness refers to the country-average score on the Cantril Ladder in the Gallup World Poll, as reported in the World Happiness Report 2018. Governance data for Figures 12.2 and 12.3 are drawn from the World Bank's World Governance Indicators, taking an average of 2014–2016 scores. Conduct of government is the mean of the scores for Government Effectiveness, Regulatory Quality, Rule of Law and Control of Corruption.

Figure 12.3 Democracy and average happiness
Gallup World Poll; World Bank. Data sources are the same as for Figure 12.2. Democratic Quality is the mean of the WGI's scores for Voice and Accountability and Political Stability/Absence of Violence.

Figure 12.4 Size of government in the OECD
World Bank. World Development Indicators, General government final consumption expenditure as percentage of GDP. Simple average of the following countries: Australia, Austria, Belgium, Canada, Denmark, Finland, France, Germany, Greece, Ireland, Israel, Italy, Japan, Luxembourg,

Netherlands, New Zealand, Norway, Portugal, Spain, Sweden, Czech Republic, United Kingdom, United States.

Figure 12.5 (*top*) Life-satisfaction in Western Europe
Eurobarometer. The question asks people: 'On the whole are you very satisfied, fairly satisfied, not very satisfied or not at all satisfied with the life you lead?' Lines refer to the simple mean of the EU-9 countries that have been in the Eurobarometer continuously since 1973. The line for 'fairly satisfied' is not shown, but equals 100 per cent minus the responses shown.

Figure 12.5 (*bottom*) Happiness in the United States
General Social Survey. The question asks respondents: 'Taken all together, how would you say things are these days – would you say that you are very happy, pretty happy, or not too happy?' The line for 'pretty happy' is not shown, but equals 100 per cent minus the responses shown.

Figure 12.6 Positive tone of the news, 1979–2010
Leetaru (2011). Figure 11 as quoted in Pinker (2018), Fig. 4.1. Units are standard deviations from the mean.

Figure 13.1 (*top*) Percentage of eighteen-year-olds spending ten or more hours per week online and percentage undertaking four face-to-face social activities
Monitoring the Future, survey of 8th, 10th, and 12th graders in the USA. See Twenge (2017), Figure 3.4.

Figure 13.1 (*bottom*) Percentage of thirteen-to eighteen-year-olds experiencing negative thoughts in last twelve months
Monitoring the Future, survey of 8th, 10th, and 12th graders in the USA. See Twenge (2017), Figure 4.5.

List of Online Annexes

Available at http://cep.lse.ac.uk/CWBH/annexesCWBH.pdf.

Notes

INTRODUCTION: THE TWO CULTURES

1. Of course some competition is fun, especially in sport and games. But in most other contexts it generates tension and fear, especially within teams and within families.
2. For a powerful argument along these lines, see Brooks (2015).
3. See Chapter 6.
4. Collier (2018).
5. Ipsos (2016). Data relate to 2016. 12 per cent had done yoga in the last month, and 28 per cent had ever done yoga. On the practice of meditation, see also Clarke et al. (2015), Table 1, which relates to 2012, and shows that 11 per cent had done deep breathing exercises and 8 per cent had meditated in the past twelve months. Comparable figures for Britain are: meditation 7 per cent in last month (youGov/University of Lancaster Survey 2013 <http://cdn.yougov.com/cumulus_uploads/document/mm7g089rhi/ YouGov-University per cent20of per cent20Lancaster-Survey-Results-Faith-Matters-130130.pdf>); yoga: 6.3 per cent in the last twelve months, 3.3 per cent in the last month. Data relate to 2015/16. (Taking Part Survey, DCMS. For data access, see <https://www.gov.uk/guidance/taking-part-survey#how-to-access-survey-data>).
6. American Psychological Association (APA) poll (2004). The survey was conducted by US market research firm Penn Schoen Berland; <https:// www.apa.org/monitor/julaug04/survey>. Comparable figures for Britain are: 28 per cent of adults have themselves visited a counsellor or a psychotherapist at some point in time; 54 per cent of people say that a family member, friend, work colleague or themselves have consulted a counsellor or psychotherapist. British Association for Counselling and Psychotherapy (BACP) Survey (2014). Poll conducted by Ipsos MORI;

<http://www.parabl.org.uk/english/wp-content/uploads/2013/11/13381_attitudes-survey-2014-key-findings.pdf>

7. Among economists the leading group has been at MIT in the Abdul Latif Jameel Poverty Action Lab (or J-PAL for short) who have already undertaken 600 randomized control trials, mostly in poor countries.

8. On the potential speed of change, see Chapter 4.

9. See Croson and Gneezy (2009) and Brdar et al. (2009).

10. For evidence that women have more other-regarding preferences than men, see results of the Gallup World Poll in Falk et al. (2018), especially Figure 3; and for evidence from surveys in seventy countries, see Schwartz & Rubel (2005). For wider reviews, see also Croson and Gneezy (2009) and Niederle (2016), who also document that women are more averse to competition between individuals. On gender differences in emotional intelligence, see, for example, Joseph and Newman (2010); Van Rooy et al. (2005); Petrides and Furnham (2000); Craig et al. (2009). Of course, it is unclear whether these differences are driven by biological or socio-historical factors. Moreover, although such gender differences have been widely shown, the magnitude of the difference is typically smaller than might be assumed from some casual stereotypes.

11. Layard (1980).

12. Obvious areas omitted include global poverty; the preservation of peace; the solution of racial and ethnic conflicts; human rights, including the advancement of women and ethnic minorities; the social care of the elderly, the disabled and the young; and animal rights.

CHAPTER 1 WHAT'S THE PURPOSE?

1. Written on 22 June 1830, and found in a friend's young daughter's birthday album. Quoted in Parekh (1993).

2. For a fuller statement of the argument, see Layard (2011), Chapter 15; de Lazari-Radek and Singer (2017) and my online Annex 1.1. Of course, not everyone accepts this argument. For example, some people would say the ultimate good is to do the will of God; but the issue still remains of what He wishes to be done. Others believe that there are multiple goods each of which are ends in themselves; but this leaves unresolved the issue of choice when different ends conflict. A related issue is whether all that matters is how people feel. Nozick (1974) asked, 'Would you plug into an experience

machine that would make you feel anything you desire, and let others do the same?' I personally would not plug in (even though I think that only experience matters) because I want to actually affect the experiences of other people. I could not do so if I was in the machine.

3. On the relative importance of reducing misery compared with increasing average happiness, see pp. 32–6, below. On minimum rights, also see p. 36.

4. 'Everybody' means people worldwide, including future generations, plus proper allowance for other sentient beings.

5. Unfortunately, the idea became known as utilitarianism, because actions were to be judged by their effects, i.e. their utility. No word worse describes an idea which aims to cultivate warmth of heart and generosity as supreme virtues. I shall use the term Happiness Principle throughout.

6. See, for example, Pinker (2018).

7. Helliwell and Wang (2012), Chapter 2.

8. For a discussion of different measures of happiness/wellbeing, see online Annex 1.2.

9. Other terms that are often used include 'flourishing', 'fulfilling' and 'quality of life'.
(1) Flourishing: for Seligman (2011) flourishing involves five different elements which spell PERMA (positive emotion, engagement, relationships, meaning and accomplishment). For Pinker (2018), flourishing involves health, happiness, freedom, knowledge, love and richness of experience (see Pinker, p.410). But, unless we know the relative importance of these different elements, the concept of flourishing is difficult to apply. Similar problems arise with the capabilities approach of Amartya Sen (1999) and Sen (2009).
(2) Fulfilling: this is fine if it means 'feeling fulfilled'. But it is often used judgementally to mean, for example, 'fulfilling your potential', which is not always a route to happiness.
(3) Quality of life: this is a good phrase, which I use liberally, especially in Chapter 8.

10. Mill's essay on Liberty is not intended as a general statement about how people should behave, but as a statement about the regulatory role of the state; see Mill (1859).

11. On such measurements, see the next note. As Annex 1.2 explains, the so-called eudaemonic methods which are currently in use bear little relation to the kind of virtue that Aristotle had in mind and that we need to find ways of measuring.

12. We know a lot about children's behaviour because we can get parents or teachers to report on them, and bad behaviour is treated as a mental illness. We know much less about the behaviour of adults, due to obvious reporting problems. We can use self-reports (e.g. measuring compassion), which are already well developed, but also records of crime, domestic violence, behaviour at work and peer-to-peer reports. To complete the picture of happiness created, we also have to place a happiness value on the kind of work people do.

13. Ricard (2015).

14. Lane (2017), Dunn et al. (2008), Aknin et al. (2012), Aknin et al. (2013), Aknin et al. (2015), Aknin et al. (2019), Otake et al. (2006). As Helliwell and Aknin et al. (2018) show on p. 10, helping behaviour gives more pleasure to the helper when it is done for the sake of the other person than when it is done for self-oriented reasons.

15. Meier and Stutzer (2008). Similarly in Japan both average altruism and average happiness rose after the 2011 earthquake – a natural experiment which presumably shows a positive effect of altruism on happiness – see Ishino et al. (2012).

16. Borgonovi (2008) and Brown et al. (2003). See also Greenfield and Marks (2004).

17. See online Annex 1.3.

18. This is broadly similar to the distribution in Germany, France and Spain, but is more equal than the distribution in the USA. See Helliwell et al. (2016), pp. 33–4.

19. For more detail, see online Annex 1.4.

20. Examples are Harsanyi (1953, 1955) and Rawls (1971). On the question in the text, they reach very different conclusions from each other and from the general case I present below. Rawls concluded that the ranking of states should be based entirely on the primary resources of the person who is least well off. This is extremely egalitarian. Harsanyi, by contrast, concludes in favour of ranking according to the average utility in the state, i.e. $\sum \Pi_i u_i$ where Π_i is the probability of being person i and u_i is the utility of person i. Harsanyi measures the utility of person i's condition as the equivalent probability of being in the best possible position and I would argue that this equivalent probability is itself a concave function of the actual happiness in condition i. See Layard (2011), p. 312.

21. If H_i is the happiness of person i, the objective of society is therefore not $\sum H_i$ but $\sum_i f(H_i)$ ($f' > 0, f'' < 0$), with $f(\ )$ more curved the more egalitarian the policy-maker. More generally, we need to include more than one

time period, and here the natural approach is to adopt the objective of $\sum_{t}\sum_{i}(1 + \delta)^{-t} f(H_{it})$ where δ is a very small discount rate. The idea here is that misery is bad, whether it happens to someone who is generally happy or to someone who is generally miserable. I agree with Bentham that policy-makers should be indifferent about the number of births and simply attempt to secure the most (weighted) happiness-years for those who are born. Thus, if a policy affects happiness *and* the number of births, we do not include in its consequences its impact on the numbers born.

Traditional additive utilitarians object to the social justice approach because it introduces individual value judgements which they claim could undermine the whole happiness approach. However, it seems wrong to impose a uniformity of view where clearly there is none.

22. On income inequality, see Chapter 11.
23. Sen (2009). On social justice, see also Sen (2017).
24. For more on this, see Layard (2011), Chapter 15. See also Anand (2016).

CHAPTER 2 WHAT MAKES PEOPLE HAPPY?

1. Moynihan and Weisman (2010).
2. Diener and Biswas-Diener (2008).
3. A. E. Clark et al. (2018).
4. Urry et al. (2004). Davidson and Begley (2012). Goleman and Davidson (2017).
5. Steptoe and Wardle (2012). The figure was privately supplied by Andrew Steptoe.
6. A. E. Clark et al. (2018), Table 16.2. See also Chapter 4 of Clark et al. (2018).
7. A. E. Clark et al. (2018), Tables 2.1 and 2.2; Stevenson and Wolfers (2008). For the best form of the function relating happiness to income, see Layard et al. (2008). In most countries the variance in income explains under 2 per cent of the variance in happiness.
8. Other factors explain up to 20 per cent of the variance. Similarly for children, family income explains under 1 per cent of the variance in emotional wellbeing at age sixteen (A. E. Clark et al. (2018), Table 10.1 and Ford et al. (2007)).
9. Suppose that in the following equation all variables are divided by their standard deviations and

$$y = \sum p_i X_i + \text{residual}$$

Then Var $(y) = 1 = \sum \sum p_i p_j X_i X_j +$ residual and the share of variance explained is $R^2 = \sum p_i^2 + \sum \sum p_i p_j r_{ij} \ (i \neq j)$ where r_{ij} is the correlation coefficient between X_i and X_j.

10. A. E. Clark et al. (2018).

11. Plomin (2018). This makes it clear that social scientists should always where possible include the relevant polygenic score in any behavioural equation. As regards the 'heritability' of happiness, there are many estimates which imply that the share of variance explained by the genes is between 30 and 60 per cent (Plomin et al. (2013), p. 322). However these estimates attribute to the genes the influence of all environmental influences (such as those in the chart) in so far as they are correlated with the genes. Nor can they handle the fact that the environment itself influences the effect of the genes.

12. This comprises some 10 per cent of the population, using the BHPS.

13. A. E. Clark et al. (2018), Table 16.1.

14. Layard (2018b), Table 2. Here misery comprises the lowest 20 per cent or so of life-satisfaction in each country.

15. Maslow (1954). In his terminology, the needs (from lowest to highest) are Physiological, Safety, Love and Belonging, Esteem, Self-actualization.

16. Tay and Diener (2011) show that, although different needs have differential impacts on happiness, the effect of satisfying each of Maslow's needs is largely independent of whether other needs have been met.

17. This does not mean that income is unimportant, as I have laid out elsewhere.

18. A. E. Clark et al. (2018), Figure 1.2.

19. A. E. Clark et al. (2018), Figure 1.5(b).

20. Helliwell and Wang (2012), Table 2.1.

21. Income inequality as such does not show up significantly in these cross-country regressions but is discussed in Chapter 11.

22. In logarithmic form.

23. World Values Survey.

24. Rojas (2018).

25. For evidence on the effect of human rights, see Diener and Diener (1995).

26. This could be pure coincidence. For example, the following model fits many of the facts. Let i be the individual and c the country.

$$\log H_{ic} = a(\log Y_{ic} - \overline{\log Y_c}) + b(\overline{\log Y_c} - \overline{\log Y_{world}})$$

with a approximately equal to b. The within-country coefficient is a, the cross-country coefficient for average happiness is b, and in the average country happiness does not rise over time.

27. Layard (2005b), p. 30, and World Happiness Report.
28. Layard et al. (2010), p. 149.
29. Easterlin et al. (2017).
30. Sacks et al. (2010), Figure 8.
31. See Helliwell, Layard and Sachs (2019), and for some countries online Annex 12.1. Overall world happiness has fallen, mainly due to a big drop in India.
32. Di Tella et al. (2003).
33. A. E. Clark et al. (2018), Table 2.4. However, if economic growth does not increase happiness, we still have to explain the country cross-section results in the table on p. 52. One consistent explanation here would be that people are comparing their country with other countries. But this is very difficult to test.
34. Sacks et al. (2010).
35. Online Annex 2.1 shows trends in each of the world's regions of stress, worry, anger, sadness and the Cantril Ladder for life evaluation.

CHAPTER 3 TRAINING OUR THOUGHTS AND FEELINGS

1. Dryden (1685).
2. For more on the themes in this chapter, see Layard and Clark (2014).
3. Wolpe (1958).
4. Paul (1966).
5. It is of course important to understand the sources of your negative thoughts and feelings (and even OK for a time to feel you are a victim). But to move forward it generally requires more than this.
6. On this paragraph, see Layard and Clark (2014).
7. Goleman (1995).
8. Seligman (2002).
9. There is also of course a long-established mystical tradition in Christianity, and increasing use of retreats and silence (as in the movement centred in Taizé, France).
10. See Williams and Penman (2011) and Williams and Kabat-Zinn (2013).
11. Kabat-Zinn (1990).
12. See Davidson et al. (2003).
13. Segal et al. (2013). Other forms of meditation have also been studied scientifically. For example, a three-month retreat focused on concentrative meditation techniques and complementary practices used to cultivate

benevolent states of mind increases telomerase activity and thus length of life. See Jacobs et al. (2011).

14. Their authors know this, and MBSR includes a final two sessions of compassion meditation (which is not mindfulness as normally conceived).

15. See, for example, Goleman (2003) and Singer and Ricard (2015).

16. A full list of these publications can be viewed on their website at <https://www.mindandlife.org/books/>.

17. T. Singer (2015) and Ricard and Singer (2017). Note that Ricard, Kabat-Zinn, Davidson and Goleman are routinely invited to the World Economic Forum in Davos.

18. Hanh (2008). See also his great book on anger, Hanh (2001).

19. Hanh and Weare (2017), p. xxxvi.

20. Shantideva (700 AD). The Bodhisattva Prayer for Humanity, written by Shantideva, an Indian Buddhist sage.

21. A remarkably uplifting and relieving experience is simply to imagine yourself inside the mind of some actual other person.

CHAPTER 4 CAN THE HAPPINESS MOVEMENT SUCCEED?

1. Twenge and Campbell (2010); Twenge (2017).

2. Twenge and Campbell (2010), p. 95.

3. Twenge (2017), Appendix Table E.2. 70 per cent of Americans think people are ruder than they were twenty years ago.

4. Twenge and Campbell (2010).

5. Collins (2001) and references therein.

6. See, for example, the strong downward trend in US crime statistics in data published by the FBI <https://ucr.fbi.gov/ucr-publications> as well as the Bureau of Justice Statistics <https://www.bjs.gov/index.cfm?ty=dcdetail&iid=245>. On other countries, see Tseloni et al. (2010). In some countries there has been an increase in violent crime in the last few years but this is not (yet at least) an established trend.

7. For a more long-term analysis of the causes of reduced violence, see Pinker (2011).

8. See references in the Introduction on gender differences in preferences.

9. See the British Social Attitudes Survey Reports published by the National Centre for Social Research; <http://www.bsa.natcen.ac.uk/latest-report/>.

10. Sometimes of course people are well advised not to interact. Women have always been subjected to unwanted attention, highlighted especially in recent years by the long-overdue #MeToo and Time's Up movements.

11. OECD (2013); Durand (2018). In the USA the data have been collected less frequently (in 2010, 2012 and 2013) in the American Time Use Survey. Data have also been collected in the Panel Study of Income Dynamics (PSID) since 2009. A USA National Academy of Sciences Panel recommends annual collection. See (Mackie and Stone (2013).

12. OECD (2016). The document did not, however, define wellbeing as subjective wellbeing.

13. The meeting was held in Paris in October 2019. In the same month (24 October) the EU Council of Ministers called on member countries and the European Commission to 'put people and their wellbeing at the centre of policy design'; <https://www.consilium.europa.eu/en/press/press-releases/2019/10/24/economy-of-wellbeing-the-council-adopts-conclusions/>.

14. In 2016 for the first time the UNDP's Human Development Report included measures of life-satisfaction.

15. Before that Bhutan and the United Arab Emirates had done the same, with formal procedures for scrutinizing all policy proposals for their impact on happiness. See UAE (2017) and Ura et al. (2012).

16. For a fuller analysis, see Durand (2018), Table 3.1, in Global Happiness Policy Report. In Germany Angela Merkel declared in 2015 that 'what matters to people must be the guideline for our policies'. So she launched a major national consultation, involving 100 meetings attended by ministers and intended to give new perspectives on what really matters; <http://www.gut-leben-in-deutschland.de/static/LB/>.

17. Stiglitz et al. (2009).

18. O'Donnell et al. (2014).

19. HM Treasury (2018).

20. Scotland has taken a lead in organizing an alliance of nations committed to wellbeing, including also New Zealand and Iceland. It is called Wellbeing Economy Governments; <http://wellbeingeconomygovs.org/>

21. See NatCen (2018); <http://natcen.ac.uk/our-research/research/british-social-attitudes>.

22. Wilson (2007) and Appiah (2011).

CHAPTER 5 EACH OF US

1. Einstein (1951).
2. In 2018, 22 per cent of Americans reported going to church every week, and a further 10 per cent almost every week. See <http://www.gallup.com/poll/1690/religion.aspx>. In many Muslim countries religious observance is also declining. For example, in Egypt the proportion of people praying five times a day has fallen from around 80 per cent in 2011 to around 60 per cent, see *The Economist* (2017).
3. US Federal Reserve Chairman, Alan Greenspan, was a long-time member of Rand's inner circle, the so-called Ayn Rand Collective (see Michael Kinsley, 'Greenspan Shrugged', *The New York Times*, 14 October 2007; <https://www.nytimes.com/2007/10/14/books/review/Kinsley-t.html>. Trump has also professed admiration for Rand, see for example an interview with Kirsten Powers in *USA Today*: <https://www.usatoday.com/story/opinion/2016/04/11/donald-trump-interview-elections-2016-ayn-rand-vp-pick-politics-column/82899566/>.
4. Dalai Lama (2012).
5. Dalai Lama (2012).
6. For some others, see p. 271 below.
7. V. King (2016). Also, for children there is V. King et al., *50 Ways to Feel Happy* (2018).
8. The Ten Keys to Happier Living align well with a number of other frameworks. These include the twelve elements identified by Sonja Lyubomirsky (2008); Martin Seligman's PERMA – positive emotion, engagement, relationships, meaning and accomplishments (Seligman (2011), and the thirteen elements identified by Seldon (2015).
9. Bullock (2000).
10. Foresight Mental Capital and Wellbeing Project (2008). The work was done by the New Economics Foundation; see <https://neweconomics.org/2008/10/five-ways-to-wellbeing-the-evidence>. See Aked et al. (2008).
11. Gottman (1994).
12. V. King (2016). See also Baumeister et al. (2001).
13. Quoted in Ricard (2015).
14. M. E. P. Seligman (2011).
15. Dolan (2014).
16. P. Gilbert (2010). There is much evidence that happy people spread happiness – happiness is contagious; see Fowler and Christakis (2008).
17. Kok et al. (2013). See also Fredrickson (2013).
18. V. King (2016) and references therein.

19. Ehrenreich (2010).
20. The calendars have already been translated by volunteers into sixteen languages.
21. Krekel et al. (2020).
22. In social science a more common measure of the effect of an intervention is its 'effect size'. This measures the change in a variable relative to its standard deviation. For changes of the size we are typically discussing in this book, the change in percentage points equals approximately forty times the 'effect size'. For example, an effect size of .25 corresponds to a change of 10 percentage points. However, this is an approximation and the numbers in the charts and tables in this book are calculated exactly.
23. The largest teaching movements are the International Positive Psychology Association (IPPA) and its offshoot the International Positive Education Network (IPEN), each with thousands of members. Teaching movements based in Britain include the School of Life, a modern humanist enterprise; and the School of Economic Science, which focuses on Eastern philosophy, and its Western counterparts, mostly pantheist. Other individual teachers with large followings include: Dan Goleman, Tal Ben-Shahar, Mo Gawdat, Gretchen Rubin, Rick Hansen and Ed Diener (with the programme called Enhance).
24. Gautier (2008).
25. On humanism, see Pinker (2018). Like many good people who have qualms about happiness, Steven Pinker uses the word 'flourishing', which he says has many dimensions. But, as we have seen, this leaves unresolved the issue of how we are to combine them. The same is true of the five elements in Seligman's PERMA; see Seligman (2011) and of the capabilities identified by Amartya Sen (2009).
26. Suppose I give $1 to a person in a poor country. And in each country happiness depends positively on own income and negatively on average income:

$$H_i = \alpha \log Y_i - \beta \log \overline{Y} + etc \quad (\alpha > \beta)$$

Then, when I give $1 to a person i in a poor country, the change in aggregate happiness in that country is:

$$\sum_j \frac{\partial H_j}{\partial Y_i} = \frac{\alpha}{Y_i} - \frac{\beta}{\overline{Y}} \frac{N}{N} = \alpha \left(\frac{1}{Y_i} - \frac{\beta}{\alpha} \frac{1}{\overline{Y}} \right)$$

This is positive if:

$$\frac{\alpha}{\beta} > \frac{Y_i}{\overline{Y}}$$

which would normally hold (with the left-hand side greater than 1 and the right-hand side smaller than 1).

And what about the change of happiness in my own country? The change of happiness when I lose $1 is positive if:

$$\frac{\alpha}{\beta} < \frac{Y_i}{\overline{Y}}$$

which might also often be true if I was reasonably well off.

On top of this the recipient in the poor country is likely to be initially less happy than the donor in the rich country (see World Happiness Report). So even if the changes summed to zero across the two countries, social justice would still call for the income transfer to be made.

27. This is inspired by the long-standing ideas of Peter Singer of Princeton University (P. Singer (2015)), and it has a strong presence at the Centre for Effective Altruism in Oxford.

28. Found online at <https://www.givewell.org/>.

29. Found online at <https://80000hours.org/>.

CHAPTER 6 TEACHERS

1. A. E. Clark et al. (2018), Chapter 1.

2. The school variable is simply a set of dummies for each school. Thus the unstandardized equation is:

$$H_i = \sum a_i X_i + \sum b_i D_{Pi} + \sum c_i D_{Si}$$

where X_i are parental characteristics, D_{Pi} are dummy variables for each primary school and D_{Si} are dummies for each secondary school. The partial correlation coefficients in the graph are the standard deviations of each right-hand term divided by the standard deviation of H.

3. A. E. Clark et al. (2018), Table 14.5.

4. Flèche (2017).

5. For the past fifty years, Phi Delta Kappa have run an influential annual poll of the American public's attitude towards public schools (see <http://pdkpoll.org/results>). In the 2017 poll, 82 per cent said it was highly important for schools to develop the interpersonal skills of pupils and 39 per cent of the respondents said it was 'extremely important' to develop skills like teamwork and persistence. This is compared to just 13 per cent

who consider standardized test scores an 'extremely important' measure of school quality. A further 82 per cent also supported more job/career skills classes, even if it had to come at the expense of time on traditional academic education.

6. Durlak et al. (2011), Hanh and Weare (2017), Adler (2016), see also Fredrickson and Branigan (2005).

7. This is an important issue. In my view a key phase, in Britain at least, is from the ages of sixteen to twenty-one. Those who argue that the early years are more crucial draw heavily on the interesting work of James Heckman, which, though suggestive, does not show conclusively that marginal investments on pre-schools have higher rates of return than at later ages (see, for example, the remarkable rates of return on apprenticeship, shown in McIntosh and Morris (2016)).

In Britain, the argument on early intervention draws heavily on the work of Feinstein (2003). This shows that children from poor homes rank higher on cognitive measures at age three than they do at age seven. However, this could simply be because some cognitive characteristics only manifest themselves at later ages (as do many psychological characteristics). On evidence for the importance of development during adolescence, see Blakemore (2018).

Interestingly one rigorous analysis took a given intervention (the Incredible Years parenting intervention) and asked whether it had better results the younger the child. The analysis found no evidence to support this hypothesis. See Gardner et al. (2019).

8. See, for example, Blanden et al. (2018).

9. Palmer (2007) and Palmer (2016). Barber and Mourshed (2007).

10. Einon et al. (1978).

11. OECD (2017). Annex 6.1 shows the country rankings for children's life-satisfaction.

12. Collishaw et al. (2004), West and Sweeting (2003), Sadler et al. (2018).
Percentage of children suffering from diagnosable mental illness in England, 2017:

Age	Boys	Girls
5–10	12.2	6.6
11–16	14.3	14.4
17–19	10.3	23.9

Source: Sadler, et al. (2018), Table 1.

13. Sadler et al. (2018).

14. McManus et al. (2016), p. 302. The figures are higher for young women than for young men.

15. Twenge et al. (2010) and Twenge (2017), Chapter 4. In 2015 over half of all US college students attended counselling for mental health concerns; see Haidt and Lukianoff (2018), p. 156.

16. On GRIT, see Duckworth (2016).

17. See <https://www.onderwijsinspectie.nl/onderwerpen/sociale-veiligheid/toezicht-op-naleving-zorgplicht-sociale-veiligheid-op-school>.

18. ISI (2017), section C.

19. The former British Prime Minister Theresa May promised that in England the government would produce a government-approved questionnaire which schools could use voluntarily. The government of South Australia already does this.

20. The Government of South Australia runs the online administration of the questionnaire and tabulation of the results. No individual is identified, but schools and classrooms are provided with benchmark data for comparison. Further information at <https://www.education.sa.gov.au/wellbeing-and-engagement-census/about-census>.

21. For some suggestions, see online Annex 6.2.

22. Below age nine it is generally found that children's replies are unreliable.

23. For wellbeing (as for academic achievement) the school should be looking at its 'value-added' – compared with a national reference norm. Some organization from outside a school should organize the measurement (typically online). In addition, the scope for gaming will be reduced if secondary schools judge themselves by how they augment pupils' wellbeing beyond the level already measured somewhere else, i.e. at primary school.

24. Hawkes (2013) and Hawkes and Hawkes (2018).

25. Bullock (2000).

26. In England, schools have a duty to promote the spiritual, moral, social and cultural development of their pupils, but without any clear guidance on what this might involve. In practice, most formal moral education happens in assemblies, or in the required weekly lesson called Religious Education.

27. Hanh and Weare (2017); Kuyken et al. (2013).

28. Durlak et al. (2011); Hale et al. (2011).

29. Hale et al. (2011).

30. Layard et al. (2018); Lordan and McGuire (2018). In most large preventative interventions, the effect-sizes are what might be considered small (here 0.18 on life-satisfaction). But the costs are small and the population affected large (see Greenberg and Abenavoli (2017)). So in this

case the estimated cost per QALY is only £1,000 compared with the critical value of around £30,000.

31. For example, the English programme of Social and Emotional Aspects of Learning (SEAL) introduced in the early 2000s was found in controlled trials in secondary schools to have no impact – largely because the teachers were not trained to use the materials. Humphrey et al. (2010).

32. Greenberg et al. (1995); Domitrovich et al. (2007); and Kam et al. (2003). In the UK the results have been somewhat less impressive, e.g. Humphrey et al. (2016). This may be because PATHS is normally being compared with the alternative of treatment-as-usual. For results of the trial in Northern Ireland, see PATHS (2013).

33. Seligman and Adler (2018).

34. Algan et al. (2013). They use data from the Civic Education Study, from the TIMMS study and from the Progress in International Reading Literacy (PIRLS) which between them allow comparisons of countries, schools and classrooms. See especially their Figure 3.

35. Elliott and Dweck (1988).

36. Webster-Stratton et al. (2011); Reinke et al. (2012); Davenport and Tansey (2009); Webster-Stratton et al. (2001); Baker-Henningham et al. (2012); Hutchings et al. (2007). For an intervention to prevent bullying, see Bonell et al. (2018).

37. Flook et al. (2013).

38. A. E. Clark et al. (2018), Table 14.4. See also Leuven and Løkken (2018) and Angrist et al. (2017).

39. Universities offering courses on wellbeing at some level or other include Northwestern, Vermont, Dartmouth, Michigan, Miami and MIT in the US, and Warwick and the London School of Economics in Britain.

40. Seldon and Martin (2017).

41. See, for example, Kessler et al. (2005).

42. Ideally mental health professionals work under supervision in a team. So the mental health service of an educational institution (if the service is small) should be part of some wider service.

43. See note 6 of this chapter.

CHAPTER 7 MANAGERS

1. E. J. Hughes (1963).

2. Krueger (2009).

3. Bryson and MacKerron (2017).

4. Jahoda (1982).

5. See Kay (1998). See also the US Business Roundtable's 'Statement on the Purpose of a Corporation' (August 2019); <https://opportunity. businessroundtable.org/wp-content/uploads/2019/09/BRT-Statement-on-the-Purpose-of-a-Corporation-with-Signatures-1.pdf>.

6. Companies Act 2006.

7. E.g. limited liability, contract enforcement, etc.

8. Edmans (2011) and Edmans (2012). For later work, see Edmans et al. (2017).

9. A. E. Clark (2001).

10. Oswald et al. (2015).

11. De Neve and Oswald (2012). Happiness is measured here by life-satisfaction. Similar results are found using positive affect measures.

12. For surveys of the evidence, see Tenney et al. (2016) and Walsh et al. (2018).

13. Deci and Ryan (2012).

14. On the value of non-financial recognition, see Ashraf et al. (2014).

15. De Neve (2018).

16. In an interesting experiment workers labelling medical images were divided into three groups. One group were told they were 'labelling tumour cells in order to assist medical researchers'; the second group were given no context for their work; and the third group were told their labels would be discarded on submission. The first group did much more work than the other two, with no loss of precision (Chandler and Kapelner (2013)). On the importance of meaning in work motivation, see also Grant (2008); Chadi et al. (2017) and Ariely et al. (2008).

17. See Chapter 2, Figure 2.2. That figure was based on data from the European Social Survey, but data from the ISSP shows a similar impact of the overall quality of work.

18. Managers also completed a self-paced computer-based course.

19. Moen et al. (2016). Voluntary quits were 7.6 per cent in the treatment group and 11.3 per cent in the control group.

20. Bloom et al. (2015), p. 167. This compares with 40 per cent in 1970.

21. Even in call-centre work there can be problems of loss of control over malpractice (where customer payouts are involved) and loss of teamwork.

22. The shift length was unchanged. Productivity rose by 9 per cent due to more minutes actively worked and it rose by 4 per cent due to more calls per minute worked.

23. The same principles apply elsewhere. For example C. Knight et al. (2010) found that care-home residents empowered to decide the decor of their

floor had improved wellbeing compared with other residents who were not empowered to do so on their floor.

24. For evidence on their effectiveness, see Blasi et al. (2008), Kruse et al. (2010) and Bryson, Clark et al. (2016).

25. On productivity, see Lazear (2000), Bloom and Van Reenen (2010) and Bandiera et al. (2017). On life-satisfaction, see Böckerman et al. (2016). Even in such cases pay based on individual performance can demotivate those who are less productive if they can compare their wages with those of others who are paid more; see Breza et al. (2017). However, this negative effect ceases when workers also know the productivity of their colleagues.

26. Bandiera et al. (2013).

27. Especially in combination with good work organization, including especially autonomy and job security. See Blasi et al. (2008). Also see Kruse et al. (2010).

28. Böckerman et al. (2016). This is with wages held constant.

29. Dahl and Pierce (2019). PRP did not include piece-work pay.

30. Card et al. (2012).

31. For example, Cohn et al. (2014) and Breza et al. (2017).

32. Barankay et al. (2012). Similarly for truck drivers, the public ranking of individual performance had a negative effect on performance once workers had received instruction in teamwork (Blader et al. (2016)). Even the ranking of teams can be counterproductive (Bandiera et al. (2013))

33. Card et al. (2012).

34. Similarly, after all Norwegian income tax records became publicly available online in 2001, the gap in happiness between rich and poor increased by 21 per cent. Bandiera et al. (2013); Perez-Truglia (2019).

35. Kellam et al. (2011).

36. Two other arguments are often brought against pay based on individually assessed performance. One is that it can distort the direction of effort. The other is that it can lead to over-arousal which can undermine performance, see online Annex 7.1.

37. World Economic Forum (WEF) (2012).

38. These can be used in-house, or businesses can hire consultants to use them and then suggest how worker wellbeing can be improved. See, for example, Robertson and Cooper (2011) and Lundberg and Cooper (2011).

39. Layard and Clark (2014); OECD (2012).

40. For example, Action for Happiness offers a two-day course called 'Doing Well from the Inside Out'. This has good before-and-after evaluation results, but without comparison to a control group.

41. Hulsheger et al. (2013).
42. See Hsieh (2012).

CHAPTER 8 HEALTH PROFESSIONALS

1. National Institute for Health and Care Excellence.
2. The World Health Organization also measures the burden of disease in terms of a similar concept: Disability-Adjusted Life Years (or DALYs).
3. A. E. Clark et al. (2018). The health measures are as described in the text except that for the UK the mental health question is 'Have you been to the doctor for an emotional problem?' and for Australia the physical health measure is the physical component of the SF36.
4. Layard (2018b), Table 2.
5. Helliwell, Layard and Sachs (2017) and Layard and Clark (2014), p. 41.
6. For UK evidence, see McManus et al. (2016). Gambling addiction is also a serious problem affecting some 0.8 per cent of adult Britons; see Conolly et al. (2017).
7. J. M. G. Williams (2001).
8. Suicide and murder figures from the Global Burden of Disease Study (2015). Battle death figures from Pinker (2011), p. 50.
9. Case and Deaton (2017). Drug overdose now costs the USA 2.8 per cent of GDP; see Council of Economic Advisers (2017) at <https://www.whitehouse.gov/sites/whitehouse.gov/files/images/The%20Underestimated%20Cost%20of%20the%20Opioid%20Crisis.pdf>.
10. For the UK we have the following percentages with any mental illness:

		1993	2014
All	16–24	13.7	17.3
	16–64	14.1	17.5
Men	16–24	8.4	9.1
	16–64	10.5	13.6
Women	16–24	19.2	26.0
	16–64	17.7	21.4

Source: McManus et al. (2016), Table 2.2. CIS-R score of 12 or more; see <https://files.digital.nhs.uk/excel/9/s/apms-2014-ch-02-tabs.xls>.

For the US we have the following percentages with any mental illness.

	2008	2017
18–25	18.5	25.8
26–49	20.7	22.2

Source: SAMHSA (2018), Figure 48; see <https://www.samhsa.gov/data/sites/default/files/cbhsq-reports/NSDUHFFR2017/NSDUHFFR2017.pdf>.

On younger adolescents in the US, see Chapter 13.

11. For more on this whole section, see Layard and Clark (2014) and Hollon et al. (2006).

12. Layard and Clark (2014), pp. 51–3.

13. This is despite the fact that the majority prefer psychological therapy (McHugh et al. (2013)).

   In the USA the proportion in treatment for depression who receive psychotherapy has fallen (see these figures from Olfson et al. (2002) and Marcus and Olfson (2010)).

	1987	1997	1998	2007
Percentage of population receiving any treatment for depression.	0.73	2.33	2.37	2.88
Percentage of those in treatment who receive:				
Psychotherapy	71.1	60.2	53.6	43.1
Medication	44.6	79.4	80.1	81.9

In the UK the proportions of people with common mental disorders receiving each type of treatment are:

Percentage of mentally ill adults who receive	2000	2007	2014
No treatment	76.9	75.6	60.6
Medication only	14.4	14.1	26.8
Counselling or therapy only	3.8	4.9	4.9
Both medication and counselling	4.8	5.5	7.7
Any counselling or therapy	8.6	10.4	12.6
Any medication	19.3	19.6	34.5
Any treatment	*23.1*	*24.4*	*39.4*

Source: McManus et al. (2016), Table 3.11.

14. Layard (2018b).
15. For example, to calculate the effects of an illness upon the quality of life (in QALYs), you have to weight the importance of five main factors (mobility, self-care, usual activities, physical pain and mental pain). The weights currently used in the British system give much less weight to mental pain than the weights obtained by regressing life-satisfaction on the five factors. See Layard and Clark (2014), pp. 65–6.
16. OECD (2012).
17. McHugh et al. (2013). See also Chilvers et al. (2001), Deacon and Abramowitz (2005) and van Schaik et al. (2004).
18. D. M. Clark (2018).
19. D. M. Clark (2018); D. M. Clark et al. (2018).
20. Parts of Norway, Sweden, Lithuania, Australia and Israel already have services, and Ontario and Quebec (both in Canada) will soon do so.
21. Andersson (2016).
22. Singla et al. (2017).
23. Kim-Cohen et al. (2003) and Kessler et al. (2005).
24. Layard and Clark (2014).
25. Layard and Clark (2014).
26. Department of Health and Social Care and Department of Education (2017).
27. Jefferson (1809): 'The care of human life and happiness, and not their destruction, is the first and only legitimate object of good government.'
28. In technical terms, it depends on the distribution of QALYs across persons, with each person's QALYs equal to the length of their lifetimes its average quality.
29. See Human Mortality Database, Period Life Table for Total Population of England and Wales. Figures refer to the standard deviation of the age of death in 1910 and 2016. If one measures the standard deviation in age of death over time, it has narrowed progressively over the time period, and continues to narrow.
30. For a different and more widely accepted definition of health inequality, see Marmot et al. (2010).
31. In Britain, the standard deviation of length of life is around 17 per cent of the average length of life; the comparable figure for life-satisfaction is around 28 per cent (in the Gallup World Poll).
32. The most striking feature of the data is that the proportional reduction in age-specific death rates has been greater at young ages. If the main factors

at work were general improvements in living standards, one might expect the effect on death rates to be similar at each age. Since this is not what we see, the changes in age-specific death rates suggest a big role for modern medicine.

33. Gawande (2014).
34. French et al. (2017), Exhibit 3.

Spending on hospital care in last 12 months of life (per cent of overall spending)

Denmark	10.0
England	14.6
France	15.0
Germany	21.2
Japan	8.2
Netherlands	8.9
Quebec	22.7
Taiwan	15.5
USA	9.9

35 Too many people die without having discussed death with their loved ones, or having exchanged feelings of gratitude, love and forgiveness.
36. As an additional feature, the new law proposed in the UK by Dignity in Dying requires that a doctor should be present when the fatal dose is taken, to ensure it works well; see the Assisted Dying Bill of 2016 which was defeated in the House of Commons.
37. Battin et al. (2007). Oregon introduced the Death with Dignity Act in 1997; California passed the End of Life Option Act in 2015. On the case for assisted dying, see Campaign for Dignity in Dying (2015).
38. For example, in Britain extra money spent on health would generate around sixty times more benefit than the corresponding cost in terms of income foregone by taxpayers (see pp. 240–41).
39. These are UK figures, from Drummond et al. (2016), p. 239, and M. Williams (2014), p. 48.
40. On the relative dangers of different substances, see Nutt (2012), Global Commission on Drug Policy (2014).
41. Nearly 1 per cent of the UK population are addicted to them; see Roberts et al. (2016), p. 266.

42. For example, the United Nations Office on Drugs and Crime (2005), Chapter 2, refers to the valuation of the illegal drug market in 2003 at $320 billion. See also Reuter and Trautmann (2009).

43. Estimates of violent deaths in Iraq since 2003 are typically under 200,000. By contrast, the following figures for intentional homicide between 2000 and 2016 relate to just five of the countries affected by violence in which drugs played a major part: Mexico, 85,000 deaths; Colombia, 281,000; the Philippines, 313,000; Guatemala, 130,000; Brazil, 821,000 (see United Nations Office on Drugs and Crime (2018) at <https://dataunodc.un.org/crime/intentional-homicide-victims>).

44. Even in the US, the prohibition of alcohol (1920-33) only applied to production and sale.

45. For heroin, the first step is to stabilize the person's life on a reducing supply of uncontaminated heroin, or a heroin substitute like methadone or buprenorphine. Where the aim is total abstinence, this can be helped by taking naltrexone to reduce craving. Once the drug situation is under control, relevant psychological therapy is crucial. For alcohol the first step is towards abstinence, which can be facilitated by taking benzodiazepines to reduce withdrawal symptoms, and other drugs like naltrexone to inhibit relapse. With alcohol addiction, psychological treatment is vital and should begin quite soon. For more on this, see Layard and Clark (2014), pp. 172-4.

46. For a description of this and policy innovations in other countries, see the Global Commission on Drug Policy (2017). When Western Australia decriminalized cannabis, there was no increase in consumption relative to other Australian states.

47. Domoslawski (2011); C. E. Hughes and Stevens (2010).

48. On Europe, see EMCDDA (2015).

49. Csete (2010).

50. Ribeaud (2004).

51. United Nations Office on Drugs and Crime (2016). The document also favours the use of evidence in policy design. See also Meacher and Warburton (2015), All Party Parliamentary Group for Drug Policy Reform, prepared for the UN General Assembly Special Session on Drugs in 2016, at which the new UN stance was adopted. More recently, the UN Chief Executive Board for Coordination have committed to 'promote alternatives to conviction and punishment in appropriate cases, including the decriminalization of drug possession for personal use, and to promote the principle of proportionality, to address prison overcrowding and

over-incarceration by people accused of drug crimes . . .' See <https://www.unsceb.org/CEBPublicFiles/CEB-2018-2-SoD.pdf>.

52. National Academies of Sciences, Engineering and Medicine (2017).

CHAPTER 9 FAMILIES

1. Rutter et al. (2010).
2. National Family and Parenting Institute (NFPI) (2000).
3. For data in the USA going back to the 1960s, see the US Census Bureau's 'Historical Living Arrangements of Adults'; at <https://www.census.gov/data/tables/timeseries/demo/families/adults.html>.
4. Ibid.
5. See US Census Bureau, Living arrangements of Children 2017; at <https://www.census.gov/data/tables/2017/demo/families/cps-2017.html>. Data is drawn from the Annual Social and Economic Supplement (ASEC) of the Current Population Survey (CPS). In 2017, 68.9 per cent of 0-to-17-year-olds were living with both parents.
6. Rosenfeld and Thomas (2012).
7. Rosenfeld and Thomas (2012), Figure 1.
8. Cacioppo et al. (2013). See also Rosenfeld (2017).
9. One concern is that an increase in 'swiping culture' may increase stress and anxiety. (An analogous point is often made in consumer psychology: there can be a 'paradox of choice' wherein a greater number of options increases stress and ultimately lowers satisfaction.)
10. For the latest official numbers in the UK, see ONS *Statistical Bulletin*: Sexual identity, UK, 2016; at <https://www.ons.gov.uk/peoplepopulationandcommunity/culturalidentity/sexuality/bulletins/sexualidentityuk/2016>.
11. Rojas (2018).
12. On the relation between child outcomes and family conflict/break-up, see A. E. Clark et al. (2015); Jekielek (1998); Hanson (1999); Amato et al. (1995); Epstein et al. (2015); A. E. Clark et al. (2018).
13. Harold and Sellers (2018). On the negative effects of easier divorce on children, see Gruber (2004). On the positive effects of easier divorce on the couple, see Stevenson and Wolfers (2006).
14. Stuart (1969); Gottman (1994), p. 57. Gottman also characterized marriages where there were five positive interactions for every one negative interaction as 'happy marriages'.

15. Baucom et al. (2015). Marriage counselling is not new, but only recently do we have interventions whose outcomes have been successfully evaluated. Note that IAPT also provides Systemic Couples Therapy based on Hewison et al. (2014).

16. Baucom et al. (1990) and Atkins et al. (2010).

17. Fischer and Baucom (2018). See also Baucom et al. (2018).

18. Epstein et al. (2015).

19. US data from Epstein et al. (2015).

20. See World Health Organization (2009) for a summary of some successful community- and school-based interventions that seek to tackle domestic violence. See also Chapter 6 above.

21. Epstein et al. (2015).

22. The difference was statistically significant – see Schulz et al. (2006), Table 3 and Figure 2. The project is called the Becoming a Family project. The Cowans also developed a successful intervention for couples whose children were beginning primary school. It lasts eighteen weeks. One set of parents are placed in groups which focus mainly on issues between the parents, while the other set are placed in groups which focus mainly on issues between the parents and the child. In a trial they were followed for ten years. For both the parents and the children, the most effective intervention was the one focused on the parents' relationship with each other. See Cowan and Cowan (2008).

23. Cowan et al. (2007). There were sixteen meetings. In the fathers' groups, as in the control group, the usual pattern emerged – people became (on average) less satisfied. The programme was called Supporting Father Involvement. The couples version has been repeated in Britain under the name the Parents as Partners programme; see Little (2016). Follow-up was after eighteen months in the USA and after six months in Britain.

24. See Acquah et al. (2017) and Harold et al. (2016).

25. Feinberg et al. (2010). There was no significant effect on the girls.

26. Bowlby (1969); Rutter et al. (2008).

27. Rutter et al. (2010).

28. Baumrind (1971).

29. Twenge and Campbell (2010).

30. Plomin (2018).

31. Layard and Mincer (1985).

32. J. Scott and Clery (2013). Women spend on average thirteen hours on housework and twenty-three hours on caring for family members each week. For men this is eight and ten hours respectively.

33. See, for example, A. E. Clark et al. (2018), Tables 11.1 and 11.3.
34. For a natural experiment, see Carneiro et al. (2015) – in Norway an increase in parental leave boosted the children's educational attainment and their wages.
35. See Eisenberg et al. (2004); Jacob et al. (2008).
36. Webster-Stratton et al. (2001). The programme is for children with mild to moderate problems. If children have severe behavioural problems, they need to be treated individually, often together with a parent. See, for example, Kazdin (2009).
37. Webster-Stratton et al. (2001).
38. See Menting et al. (2013) for a meta-analysis.
39. That is, 'oppositional defiant disorder'. See S. Scott et al. (2014). Anti-social character traits were also reduced, and emotions expressed by the parents were warmer.
40. Layard and Clark (2014).
41. Other well-evidenced courses of parent training include the so-called 'Triple P' programme – the Positive Parenting Program.

CHAPTER 10 COMMUNITIES

1. From Martin Luther King Jr.'s lecture, 11 December 1964, to mark his acceptance of the Nobel Peace Prize; at <https://www.nobelprize.org/prizes/peace/1964/king/lecture/>.
2. TNS Loneliness Omnibus Survey for Age UK (April 2014). For people over sixty-five the figure is 1 million.
3. Steptoe and Lassale (2018), Figures 9.2 and 9.3.
4. McDaid et al. (2017), p. 32.
5. Holt-Lunstad et al. (2010); Holt-Lunstad et al. (2015).
6. See Figures 7.1 and 7.2.
7. Helliwell and Wang (2011), Table 3, shows clearly how strongly in Canada life-satisfaction depends on the sense of belonging to your community, your province and your country, and on your trust in your neighbours and co-workers.
8. For time devoted to these activities, see Krueger et al. (2009) and Gershuny and Halpin (1996).
9. Putnam (2007) describes social capital as 'features of social life – networks, norms and trust – that enable participants to act together more effectively to pursue shared objectives'. These objectives must, in my view, include the

sheer pleasure of being together. For evidence that social capital increases happiness, see Putnam (2000), Section IV. On social capital, see also Halpern (2004, 2015).

10. People underestimate the trustworthiness of others; see Helliwell and Wang (2011).

11. In Britain about one third of the income of NGOs comes from public funds; see Hall (1999).

12. Brown et al. (2003). Needless to say we want volunteers to volunteer because they want to help – not because it looks good on a CV. A sad example of the latter is the flyer for the LSE Careers Centre with the rhyme 'Boost Your Career, Volunteer'.

13. Tan et al. (2006).

14. Carlson et al. (2015).

15. McDaid et al. (2017).

16. Pitkala et al. (2009). The costs of health care per person per year were €1,522 in the experimental treatment group compared with €2,465 in the control group. This statistically significant difference was larger than the total cost of the intervention (€881 including the group rehab and the programme costs, transport, food and the training and tutoring of the group leaders).

17. Through time-use surveys, the OECD estimates the economic value of volunteering for Germany in 2013 to be around USD 118 billion, or 3.3 per cent of real GDP. See Table 5.4 in OECD (2015). The figure is roughly comparable in other countries like the UK (2.5 per cent) and the USA (3.7 per cent).

18. Lawlor et al. (2014). Note that just visiting lonely people is often not particularly effective.

19. Halpern (2010), Figure 2.1.

20. Dustmann and Fasani (2016).

21. Halpern (2010).

22. Leong (2010).

23. Singleton et al. (1998), Table 12.1.

24. Barnoski and Aos (2004).

25. Oesterle et al. (2018).

26. Bentham (1789).

27. Putnam (2007); Alesina and La Ferrara (2000); Alesina and La Ferrara (2002); Alesina and Glaeser (2004); Glaeser et al. (2000).

28. Langella and Manning (2016). See also Longhi (2014), who finds that this result applies only to the white British population. However, if we look only at the effects of immigrants coming from Eastern Europe, Ivlevs and

Veliziotis (2018) find that life-satisfaction is actually increased for residents who are younger or employed or on higher incomes, and reduced for people who are older or unemployed or on lower incomes.

29. Akay et al. (2014).

30. Betz and Simpson (2013).

31. Helliwell, Layard and Sachs (2018), p. 39.

32. Many studies have failed to find significant average effects on wages or employment, but there are clear individual instances of such effects. These can create great resentment both among those affected and also often in areas of very low immigration.

33. Helliwell, Huang, Wang and Shiplett (2018), p. 35.

34. Rao (2019).

35. There is a huge literature on whether people are happier living in villages or towns/cities of different sizes. But it is so far inconclusive.

36. Around London, land in the Green Belt with no special amenity value and within 800 metres of a tube or train station would be able to accommodate 1 million homes; see Stringer (2014).

37. See the minutes of the All Parliamentary Policy Group on Wellbeing Economics meeting, held on 12 June 2014: at <https://wellbeingeconomics. wordpress.com/2014/06/10/meeting-4-planning-transport-and-well-being/>. This is not atypical: most government departments have somewhat arbitrary and unrelated targets.

38. For a pioneering controlled study of the wellbeing effects of an urban improvement scheme, see Anderson et al. (2017).

39. For more on the Copenhagen project, see Gehl and Gemzøe (2004); Gehl and Rogers (2010).

40. Richard et al. (2008).

41. Gehl (2011). See also Whyte (1980).

42. Cohen and Spacapan (1984).

43. Halpern (1995).

44. Gifford (2007).

45. Office for National Statistics (2016). Living in high-rise compared with terraced housing reduced life-satisfaction by 0.3 points. In a study in the USA, more space was good for wellbeing but only when measured relative to the space which others had; see Bellet (2017).

46. See for example Davies-Cooper et al. (2014) and Vartanian et al. (2015).

47. Krekel et al. (2016).

48. 0.007 x 6,000. See Krekel et al. (2016). For a similar estimate, see White et al. (2013).

49. Life-satisfaction (LS) = 0.3 *log income* (Y) + *etc*. Thus

$$\Delta LS = \frac{0.3}{Y}\Delta Y \text{ and } \frac{\Delta Y}{ALS} = \frac{Y}{0.3}$$

50. Holding a constant distance from the city centre.

51. White et al. (2013). See also Alcock et al. (forthcoming).

52. Ulrich (1984).

53. Montgomery (2013).

54. Kuo and Sullivan (2001).

55. Weinstein et al. (2009).

56. MacKerron and Mourato (2013). See also Testoni and Dolan (2018).

57. Montgomery (2013), p. 110.

58. See Rajan (2019) and Collier (2018).

CHAPTER 11 ECONOMISTS

1. Ben Bernanke at the 32nd General Conference of the International Association for Research in Income and Wealth, Cambridge, Massachusetts; at <https://www.federalreserve.gov/newsevents/speech/bernanke20120806a.htm>.

2. This was the way economists framed their objective up till the 1930s. After that they redefined 'utility' in terms of preference-satisfaction, but, as I shall show, it needs to revert to its earlier meaning.

3. A slightly better measure of income is Net National Income, but this is less commonly used.

4. I was also shocked by the way economics textbooks like *The Theory of Price* by George Stigler discussed policy conclusions without having discussed welfare economics. Layard and Walters (1978) tried to rectify this.

5. Layard et al. (2008).

6. See, for example, Layard and Glaister (1994).

7. See Layard and Glaister (1994).

8. Quality is measured on a scale of 0–1. For some problems with QALYs, see Layard and Clark (2014), pp. 188–90.

9. For a detailed analysis, see Layard and O'Donnell (2015).

10. This unethical procedure is usually justified by the so-called Hicks/Kaldor criterion, which says that if the gainers could compensate the losers there is a net improvement, even if no compensation is paid. No ethical justification for the rule has ever been provided. A dreadful example of the

use of this criterion is the analysis done to justify a new high-speed rail link from London to the North of England (HS2).

11. Durand (2018). The UAE approach is the most all-embracing, see UAE (2017). For the UK's new Green Book, see HM Treasury (2018), paragraphs 2.3, 4.15, 4.16, 6.21 and 6.22.

12. Lucas (2003).

13. A. E. Clark et al. (2018), Tables 4.2 and 5.2. Data for the UK.

14. See Kahneman (2011), De Neve et al. (2018) and Boyce et al. (2013) – the last two for confirmation from real-world time series using happiness data at the country- and individual-level respectively.

15. See Layard et al. (2012), which summarizes the controversy between Easterlin (2010), Chapter 5, and Sacks et al. (2010).

16. In addition, people also adapt to higher levels of income. But this is generally a less important factor; see A. E. Clark et al. (2008) and A. E. Clark et al. (2018), Chapter 2. See also Vendrik (2013).

17. Baumol (1967).

18. This is also one of the advantages of immigration.

19. A. E. Clark et al. (2018), Table 16.2.

20. Layard and Nickell (2011).

21. To our great satisfaction, the explanation we gave for unemployment up to 1990 worked equally well in explaining unemployment in different European countries between 1990 and 2002; see 'Introduction to New Edition' in Layard et al. (2005).

22. A. E. Clark et al. (2018), pp. 74 and 63, show that one standard deviation of job quality raises life-satisfaction by 0.4 points, while unemployment lowers it by 0.7 points. So if it were better for a person to remain unemployed than to accept a job, the job would need to be very bad relative to the one they could get by waiting.

23. See, for example,. Knabe et al. (2017), which finds 'workfare' participants have a level of life-satisfaction above that of those who are left unemployed (though lower than that of employed workers).

24. Layard and Philpott (1991).

25. Layard (2000), Blundell et al. (2004).

26. Marlow et al. (2012), p. 70.

27. Layard and Nickell (2011).

28. This should be automatic, but with a right for the client to opt out.

29. Autor et al. (2013).

30. Acemoglu and Autor (2011); Acemoglu and Autor (2012). Foreign trade has a major impact on the pattern of jobs (Autor et al. (2013)) but is not the main influence on increased wage inequality.

31. For Britain, see McIntosh and Morris (2016) and Walker and Zhu (2013).
32. For early analyses of the race between the demand for skill and the supply of skill, see Jackman et al. (1999) and Manacorda and Petrongolo (1999).
33. OECD data.
34. This both reduces the number of unskilled people and makes them scarcer, thus raising their wages.
35. Thomas and Dimsdale (2017), version 3.1.
36. This argument relates to an ongoing situation. If the degree of redistribution is increased at some time, we have also to take into account the extra cost due to loss aversion.
37. Atkinson and Stiglitz (1980).
38. Layard (1980); Layard (2005a); Layard (2006).
39. See Kahneman (2011), Thaler and Sunstein (2008), and Thaler (2015).
40. For example, Haushofer and Shapiro (2016) report on an unconditional cash-transfer trial in Kenya. For the 'large transfer group' their monthly income increased by a factor of three and their life-satisfaction increased by 0.36 standard deviations. The cost was high relative to the benefit in terms of wellbeing.
41. At present this means the respondent is in the bottom 10 per cent of the adult population.
42. This calculation of cost ignores the savings which flow back from reduced mental illness.
43. Wilkinson and Pickett (2009), Wilkinson and Pickett (2018).
44. Wilkinson and Pickett (2008), Wilkinson and Pickett (2018). On mental illness, the Kessler data which they use are very weakly correlated with the WHO estimate in World Health Organization (2017).
45. Both indirectly and directly. The direct effects would be attributable to diminishing marginal utility of income. Doubtless this effect exists, but it is too small to be detected. For example, if $H_i = 0.3 \log y_i$, then the difference in average happiness between Sweden and the USA on account of the differences in income equality would be roughly 0.075 points (out of 10). To derive this, we use a Taylor's series expansion. So if $H_i = 0.3 \log y_i$ and π_i is the frequency of income y_i, then

$$\overline{H} = 0.3 \sum_i \pi_i \log y_i = 0.3 \sum_i \pi_i \left(\log \overline{y} + \frac{1}{\overline{y}}(y_i - \overline{y}) - \frac{1}{2\overline{y}^2}(y_i - \overline{y})^2 \right)$$
$$= 0.3 \log \overline{y} - 0.15 \frac{SD^2(y)}{\overline{y}^2}$$

We assume $SD(y) / \overline{y} = 0.4$ in Sweden and 0.8 in the US.

46. See, for example, Goff et al. (2018), who find small or insignificant effects. For an earlier exploration of this issue, see Stevenson and Wolfers (2010).

47. Goff et al. (2018). A one-point increase in the standard deviation of happiness is associated with an increase in average happiness of 1 point (out of 10).

48. Goff et al. (2018). Table 6 shows that the relation between social trust and happiness inequality is closer than between social trust and income inequality.

49. Layard (2018b).

50. Easterlin (2010), Figures 5.3 and 5.4.

51. Easterlin et al. (2017).

52. Easterlin et al. (2017).

53. Knight and Gunatilaka (2018).

54. Tay and Diener (2011).

55. Only 10 per cent of migrants are refugees and, due to small sample numbers, the report includes migrants of all sorts in a single analysis.

56. If there is a flow of migrants between any two countries, the migrants gain in happiness nearly 90 per cent of the difference in happiness between the two countries.

57. Helliwell, Huang, Wang and Shiplett (2018), p. 35.

58. Helliwell, Layard and Sachs (2018), p. 9.

59. Collier (2013).

60. The Happiness Principle requires that we adopt many lower-level rules of thumb, which we generally respect (Hare (1981)). These include the rights of a country's residents to control entry to their country, except in the case of refugees.

61. See, for example, my address at the American Economic Association meetings in 2018; Layard (2018a).

CHAPTER 12 POLITICIANS AND PUBLIC SERVANTS

1. Jefferson (1809).

2. For other similar arguments, see Bok (2011) and Diener et al. (2009).

3. Ward (2015; forthcoming). The explanatory variables also included average income, the unemployment rate, the inflation rate (all three insignificant), as well as the share of the governing parties at the previous election, a fixed effect per country, and a fixed effect per year. All variables were standardized using their standard deviations over the whole sample of

countries and elections. If a different regression is run where variables are standardized using their standard deviations in each country, the partial correlations for life-satisfaction and economic growth are equal in size. In a separate analysis, greater individual life-satisfaction increases the probability of an individual supporting the government. On this, see also Liberini, Redoano and Proto (2017).

4. Ward et al. (2019). See also Ward (2019). The explanatory variables include the average share of the vote for the Republican Party in the previous four presidential elections.

5. 'Eventually, the poor woman's mother-in-law solved the problem by promising to pawn a set of gold earrings and so Nasam Velankanni got to hold her newborn baby.' See Holmberg and Rothstein (2011).

6. Norris (2003), Table 2.

7. Helliwell, Huang, Grover and Wang (2018). One hundred and fifty-seven countries were surveyed. Fixed effects are included in the analysis. See also Ott (2011).

8. See Helliwell, Huang, Grover and Wang (2018). But this controls for many variables which may themselves be affected by democracy.

9. There was a reform in 2007, but it was evolutionary not revolutionary, see Zhang and Oyama (2016).

10. Franks and Mayer (1996); Bruner (2002). However, the shareholders of the company which is bought do on average gain, even though their workers usually lose.

11. Ipsos MORI (2017), p. 55.

12. For example in the British Rhine Army huge prestige went to the troop which was the very first to range on to an Army target.

13. This statement is less true in some developing countries. For an assessment of the effects of privatization in Britain, see Bishop and Kay (1989).

14. See O'Neill (2002).

15. Syed (2015).

16. Hagen (2015); EUROCONTROL (2006).

17. Aviation Safety Network.

18. Blair (2010), p. 216.

19. *The Economist* (2018).

20. On economic growth and public spending, there is a large and inconclusive literature, see Nijkamp and Poot (2004).

21. Flavin et al. (2011), Table 1, Column 2. Data from World Values Survey.

22. This is provided the technical quality of government is good enough. Using data for 130 nations from the Gallup World Poll, Ott (2011) confirms these

results. Similar results were also found in Alvarez-Diaz et al. (2010) for a cross-section of US states, using the DDB Lifestyle Survey.

23. Using Gallup World Poll data on 106 countries, we regressed average happiness on average log GDP and (separately) (a) the share of tax in GDP, (b) the share of government services in GDP, and (c) the share of welfare spending in GDP. In none of the three cases did tax/spending have any significant effect in the equation. For all of our measures, we averaged the data over the three-year period between 2014 and 2016.

24. On the role of social comparisons, see Layard et al. (2010).

25. Suppose $LS = 0.3 \log Y$ and income is £30,000. Then
$$\frac{\partial LS}{\partial Y} = \frac{0.3}{Y} = \frac{0.3}{30,000} = \frac{1}{100,000}$$ So if £15,000 is raised in small amounts from many people, $\Delta LS = \left(\frac{\partial LS}{\partial Y}\right).15,000 = 0.15$. This ignores the role of comparator income.

26. Claxton et al. (2015) estimate that the spending of £15,000 in today's money generates one extra Quality Adjusted Life Year where quality is measured on a scale of 0–1. But life-satisfaction is measured on a scale of 0–10, so we can roughly equate 1 QALY to 10 life-satisfaction years; see Peasgood et al. (2018).

27. Some people argue that higher taxes will reduce private charitable giving. The evidence here is ambiguous; see Bredtmann (2016).

28. Populism can be defined in different ways, but is typically characterized by a strong anti-establishment view, often combined with nationalist sentiment, see Mudde (2007).

29. There is tentative evidence that those supporting Brexit are less contented than other citizens (e.g. Liberini, Oswald, Proto and Redoano (2017)).

30. Data on individual European countries are in online Annex 12.1. Since 2006, when these data were first collected in the Gallup World Poll, there has been a rise in negative emotion (average of anger, worry and sadness) experienced the previous day and a decline in positive emotion (average of happiness, laughter and enjoyment) in Western Europe; see Helliwell, Huang and Wang (2019). See also online Annex 2.1.

31. For a summary of the evidence that news of bad events generally attracts more interest than good events, see Baumeister et al. (2001). See also Marshall and Kidd (1981).

32. Leetaru (2011). Data is taken from *Summary of World Broadcasts,* which tracks newspaper articles, conference proceedings, television and radio broadcasts, periodicals and non–classified technical reports in their native languages in over 130 countries.

33. Pinker (2018).
34. Lewis (2010); M. A. King (2016).
35. The Federal Communications Commission (FCC) fairness doctrine was introduced in 1949.
36. Even among professional academic economists this is also the case. A recent study showed a shocking amount of abusive language and behaviour on the Economics Job Market Rumors forum for economists, on which people post anonymously; see Wu (2018).
37. Murthy and Lakshminarayana (2006).
38. Pinker (2011).
39. Haidt and Lukianoff (2018), p. 58.
40. An egregious error occurred when Tony Blair sacked Home Secretary Charles Clark for a long-standing failure of the Home Office to deport immigrants convicted of crimes, after their release from prison. This happened to come to light when he was Home Secretary.

CHAPTER 13 SCIENTISTS AND TECHNOLOGISTS

1. Bacon (1597).
2. We may also need new ways to extract carbon dioxide from the atmosphere.
3. D. King, Browne et al. (2015).
4. Mazzucato (2015).
5. By 2050 Britain has committed to reduce emissions to no higher than 20 per cent of their level in 1990.
6. D. King, Browne et al. (2015).
7. It is run by the annual meeting of Energy Ministers of the member countries and a seven-person international secretariat. It has seven working parties on the different technological challenges.
8. This situation could only be avoided if cost-effective ways are discovered for extracting carbon dioxide from the atmosphere.
9. D. King, Schrag et al. (2015).
10. The British government uses a discount rate of 3.5 per cent. Of this, 2 per cent is due to higher income, on the basis that the marginal utility of income is inversely proportional to income, so that a forecast 2 per cent growth rate per annum makes next year's marginal pound sterling worth 2 per cent less in happiness than this year's pound. The remaining

1.5 per cent is due to 'catastrophic risk and pure time preference'. A 3.5 per cent discount rate means that £1 in fifty years' time is worth only 17 pence today.

11. Unless one assumes pure time preference – for which there is no obvious ethical justification.

12. See ranking of countries in Helliwell, Layard and Sachs (2018).

13. We are now at roughly 1 degree Celsius above pre-industrial temperatures, and the current rate of warming is 0.2 degrees per decade (IPCC (2018)).

14. United Nations Environment Programme (2018).

15. For example, these gadgets may well include deep brain stimulation for conditions like depression, Parkinson's disease and dystonia; see Perlmutter and Mink (2006).

16. Also, perhaps, deep brain stimulation and transcranial magnetic stimulation.

17. Kramer (1994).

18. Currently in Britain, if a public body considers that parents' choices risk harming a child, it can challenge them in court. Doctors and social workers can ask a judge for an order to override the legal state of parental responsibility.

19. Plomin (2018); see also Okbay et al. (2016).

20. For parents with fertility problems, we already allow IVF to fertilize many eggs and choose the one most free of disease.

21. See Layard et al. (1994). This explains why unemployment fluctuates with aggregate demand but is not generally trended.

22. See Twenge (2017). Monthly active users of Facebook went from 250 million in 2009 to 500 million in 2010 and then in a straight line to 2 billion in 2017.

23. Tromholt (2016). Lonely: 16 per cent versus 25 per cent; depressed: 22 per cent versus 35 per cent. See also Deters and Mehl (2013).

24. Shakya and Christakis (2017); Kross et al. (2013).

25. Haidt and Lukianoff (2018).

26. An example would be to ban all anonymous writing.

27. Schools which ban the carrying of mobile phones in school achieve better results; see Beland and Murphy (2016).

CONCLUSION: ACTIONS FOR HAPPINESS

1. See Chapter 6.

A NOTE OF THANKS

1. O'Donnell et al. (2014).

References

Acemoglu, D., and Autor, D. (2011). Skills, tasks and technologies: implications for employment and earnings, *Handbook of Labor Economics*, Vol. 4B, pp. 1043–171. San Diego, CA: Elsevier.

Acemoglu, D., and Autor, D. (2012). What does human capital do? A review of Goldin and Katz's *The Race between Education and Technology*, *Journal of Economic Literature*, 50(2), 426–63.

Acquah, D., Sellers, R., Stock, L., and Harold, G. (2017). *Inter-parental Conflict and Outcomes for Children in the Contexts of Poverty and Economic Pressure.* London: Early Prevention Foundation.

Adler, A. (2016). *Teaching Well-being increases Academic Performance: Evidence from Bhutan, Mexico, and Peru.* University of Pennsylvania, Publicly Accessible Penn Dissertations (1572).

Akay, A., Constant, A., and Giulietti, C. (2014). The impact of immigration on the well-being of natives, *Journal of Economic Behavior & Organization*, 103(C), 72–92.

Aked, J., Marks, N., Cordon, C., and Thompson, S. (2008). *Five Ways to Well-being: The evidence.* London: New Economics Foundation.

Aknin, L. B., Hamlin, J. K., and Dunn, E.W. (2012). Giving leads to happiness in young children, *PLOS ONE*, 7(6), e39211.

Aknin, L. B., Barrington-Leigh, C., Dunn, E., Helliwell, J., Burns, J., Biswas-Diener, R., Kemeza, I., Nyende, P., Ashton-James, C., and Norton, M. (2013). Prosocial spending and well-being: cross-cultural evidence for a psychological universal, *Journal of Personality and Social Psychology*, 104(4), 635–52.

Aknin, L. B., Broesch, T., Hamlin, J., and Van de Vondervoot, J. (2015). Prosocial behavior leads to happiness in a small-scale rural society, *Journal of Experimental Psychology: General*, 144 (4), 788–95.

Aknin, L. B., Whillans, A. V., Norton, M. I., and Dunn, E.W. (2019). Happiness and prosocial behavior: an evaluation of the evidence, in Helliwell,

Layard and Sachs (eds), *World Happiness Report 2019*. New York: Columbia University, SDSN.

Alcock, I., White, M., Wheeler, B., Fleming, L., and Depledge, M. (forthcoming). Longitudinal effects on mental health of moving to greener and less green urban areas, *Environmental Science and Technology*.

Alesina, A., and Glaeser, E. (2004). *Fighting Poverty in the US and Europe: A world of difference.* Oxford: Oxford University Press.

Alesina, A., and La Ferrara, E. (2000). Participation in heterogeneous communities, *The Quarterly Journal of Economics*, 115(3), 847–904.

Alesina, A., and La Ferrara, E. (2002). Who trusts others? *Journal of Public Economics*, 85(2), 207–34.

Algan, Y., Cahuc, P., and Shleifer, A. (2013). Teaching practices and social capital, *American Economic Journal: Applied Economics*, 5(3), 189–210.

Alvarez-Diaz, A., Gonzalez, L., and Radcliff, B. (2010). The politics of happiness: on the political determinants of quality of life in the American states, *The Journal of Politics*, 72(3), 894–905.

Amato, P. R., Loomis, L. S., and Booth, A. (1995). Parental divorce, marital conflict, and offspring well-being during early adulthood, *Social Forces*, 73(3), 895–915.

Anand, P. (2016). *Happiness, Well-being and Human Development: The case for subjective measures*, UNDP Human Development Report – Background Paper. New York: United Nations Development Programme (UNDP).

Anderson, J., Ruggeri, K., Steemers, K., and Huppert, F. (2017). Lively social space, well-being activity, and urban design: findings from a low-cost community-led public space intervention, *Environment and Behavior*, 49(6), 685–716.

Andersson, G. (2016). Internet-delivered psychological treatments, *Annual Review of Clinical Psychology*, 12, 157–79.

Angrist, J. D., Lavy, V., Leder-Luis, J., and Shany, A. (2017). *Maimonides Rule Redux*, NBER Working Papers 23486. Cambridge, MA: National Bureau of Economic Research.

Appiah, K. A. (2011). *The Honor Code: How moral revolutions happen.* New York: W. W. Norton.

Ariely, D., Kamenica, E., and Prelec, D. (2008). Man's search for meaning: the case of Legos, *Journal of Economic Behavior and Organization*, 67(3–4), 671–77.

Ashraf, N., Bandiera, O., and Jack, B. K. (2014). No margin, no mission? A field experiment on incentives for public service delivery, *Journal of Public Economics*, 120, 1–17; doi: https://doi.org/10.1016/j.jpubeco.2014.06.014.

Atkins, D. C., Marín, R. A., Lo, T. T., Klann, N., and Hahlweg, K. (2010). Outcomes of couples with infidelity in a community-based sample of couple therapy, *Journal of Family Psychology*, 24(2), 212.

Atkinson, A. B., and Stiglitz, J. E. (1980). *Lectures on Public Economics*. Maidenhead: McGraw-Hill.

Autor, D., Dorn, D., and Hanson, G. H. (2013). The China syndrome: local labor market effects of import competition in the United States, *American Economic Review*, 103(6), 2121–68.

Bacon, F. (1597). *Meditationes sacrae* (Religious meditations): Of Heresies, 'knowledge is power'. London.

Baker-Henningham, H., Scott, S., Jones, K., and Walker, S. (2012). Reducing child conduct problems and promoting social skills in a middle-income country: cluster randomised controlled trial, *British Journal of Psychiatry*, 201, 101–8.

Bandiera, O., Barankay, I., and Rasul, I. (2013). Team incentives: evidence from a firm level experiment, *Journal of the European Economic Association*, 11(5), 1079–1114; doi: 10.1111/jeea.12028.

Bandiera, O., Fischer, G., Prat, A., and Ytsma, E. (2017). *Do Women Respond Less to Performance Pay? Building evidence from multiple experiments*. CEPR Discussion Paper (11724). London: Centre for Economic Policy Research.

Barankay, I. et al. (2012). *Rank Incentives: Evidence from a randomized workplace experiment*, Working Paper, Business Economics and Public Policy Papers, 7 July: at < https://repository.upenn.edu/bepp_papers/75>.

Barber, M., and Mourshed, M. (2007). *How the World's Best-Performing School Systems Come Out on Top*. New York: McKinsey & Company.

Barnoski, R., and Aos, S. (2004). *Outcome evaluation of Washington State's Research-based Programs for Juvenile Offenders*. Olympia, WA: Washington State Institute for Public Policy, 460.

Battin, M. P., Van der Heide, A., Ganzini, L., Van der Wal, G., and Onwuteaka-Philipsen, B. D. (2007). Legal physician-assisted dying in Oregon and the Netherlands: evidence concerning the impact on patients in 'vulnerable' groups, *Journal of Medical Ethics*, 33(10), 591–7.

Baucom, D. H., Sayers, S. L., and Sher, T. G. (1990). Supplementing behavioral marital therapy with cognitive restructuring and emotional expressiveness training: an outcome investigation, *Journal of Consulting and Clinical Psychology*, 58(5), 636.

Baucom, D. H., Epstein, N. B., Kirby, J. S., and LaTaillade, J. J. (2015). Cognitive-behavioral couple therapy, in A. Gurman, J. Lebow and D. Snyder (eds.), *Clinical Handbook of Couple Therapy*, 5th edn. New York: Guilford Press, pp. 23–60.

Baucom, D. H., Fischer, M. S., Worrell, M., Corrie, S., Belus, J. M., Molyva, E., and Boeding, S. E. (2018). Couple-based intervention for depression: an effectiveness study in the National Health Service in England, *Family Process*, 57(2), 275–92.

Baumeister, R. F., Bratslavsky, E., Finkenauer, C., and Vohs, K. D. (2001). Bad is stronger than good, *Review of General Psychology*, 5(4), 323.

Baumol, W. J. (1967). Macroeconomics of unbalanced growth: the anatomy of urban crisis, *The American Economic Review*, 57(3), 415–26.

Baumrind, D. (1971). Current patterns of parental authority, *Developmental Psychology*, 4(1p2), 1.

Beland, L.-P., and Murphy, R. (2016). Ill communication: technology, distraction and student performance, *Labour Economics*, 41, 61–76.

Bellet, C. (2017). *The Paradox of the Joneses: Superstar houses and mortgage frenzy in suburban America*, CEP Discussion Paper (CEPDP 1462). Centre for Economic Performance, LSE.

Bentham, J. (1789). *An Introduction to the Principles of Morals and Legislation*, J. H. Burns and H. L. A. Hart (eds.). Oxford: Oxford University Press, 1996.

Betz, W., and Simpson, N. (2013). The effects of international migration on the well-being of native populations in Europe, *IZA Journal of Migration*, 2(1), 1–21.

Bishop, M. R., and Kay, J. A. (1989). Privatization in the United Kingdom: lessons from experience, *World Development*, 17(5), 643–57.

Blader, S., Gartenberg, C., and Prat, A. (2016). *The Contingent Effect of Management Practices*, CEPR Discussion Paper (11057). London: Centre for Economic Policy Research.

Blair, T. (2010). *A Journey*. London: Hutchinson.

Blakemore, S. J. (2018). *Inventing Ourselves: The secret life of the teenage brain*. London: Doubleday.

Blanden, J., Del Bono, E., Hansen, K., McNally, S., and Rabe, B. (2018). Nursery attendance and children's outcomes, *CentrePiece*, 23(1) (CEPCP 524). Centre for Economic Performance, LSE.

Blasi, J., Freeman, R., Mackin, C., and Kruse, D. (2008). *Creating a Bigger Pie? The effects of employee ownership, profit sharing, and stock options on workplace performance*, NBER Working Papers 14230. Cambridge, MA: National Bureau of Economic Research.

Bloom, N., and Van Reenen, J. (2010). Why do management practices differ across firms and countries? *Journal of Economic Perspectives*, 24(1), 203–24. doi: 10.1257/jep.24.1.203.

Bloom, N., Liang, J., Roberts, J., and Ying, Z.J. (2015). Does working from home work? Evidence from a Chinese experiment, *The Quarterly Journal of Economics*, 130(1), 165–218. doi: 10.1093/qje/qju032.

Blundell, R., Dias, M. C., Meghir, C., and Van Reenen, J. (2004). Evaluating the employment impact of a mandatory job search program, *Journal of the European Economic Association*, 2(4), 569–606.

Böckerman, P., Bryson, A., Kauhanen, A., and Kangasniemi, M. (2016). *Does Job Support Make Workers Happy?*, Working Paper No. 16-16. Department of Quantitative Social Science-UCL Institute of Education, University College London.

Bok, D. (2011). *The Politics of Happiness: What government can learn from the new research on well-being*. Princeton, NJ: Princeton University Press.

Bonell, C., Allen, E., Warren, E., McGowan, J., Bevilacqua, L., Jamal, F., Legood, R., Wiggins, M., Opondo, C., and Mathiot, A. (2018). Effects of the Learning Together intervention on bullying and aggression in English secondary schools (inclusive): a cluster randomised controlled trial, *The Lancet*, 392(10163), 2452–64.

Borgonovi, F. (2008). Doing well by doing good: the relationship between formal volunteering and self-reported health and happiness, *Social Science and Medicine*, 66(11), 2321–34.

Bowlby, J. (1969). *Attachment and Loss*, Vol. 1: *Attachment*. London: Hogarth Press and Institute of Psychoanalysis.

Boyce, C., Wood, A., Banks, J., Clark, A. E., and Brown, G. (2013). Money, well-being, and loss aversion: does an income loss have a greater effect on well-being than an equivalent income gain?, *Psychological Science*, 24(12), 2557–62.

Bradford, A. C., Bradford, W. D., Abraham, A., and Adams, G. B. (2018). Association between US state medical cannabis laws and opioid prescribing in the Medicare Part D population, *JAMA Internal Medicine*, 178(5), 667–72.

Brdar, I., Rijavec, M., and Miljković, D. (2009). Approaches to happiness, life goals and wellbeing, in T. Freire (ed.), *Understanding Positive Life: Research and practice on positive psychology*. Lisbon: Climepsi Editores, pp. 45–64.

Bredtmann, J. (2016). Does government spending crowd out voluntary labor and donations?, *IZA World of Labor*, January.

Breza, E., Kaur, S., and Shamdasani, Y. (2017). The morale effects of pay inequality, *The Quarterly Journal of Economics*, 133(2), 611–63.

Brooks, D. (2015). *The Road to Character*. London: Penguin Books.

Brown, S. L., Nesse, R. M., Vinokur, A. D., and Smith, D. M. (2003). Providing social support may be more beneficial than receiving it: results from a prospective study of mortality, *Psychological Science*, 14(4), 320–27.

Bruner, R. F. (2002). Does M & A pay? A survey of evidence for the decision-maker, *Journal of Applied Finance*, 12(1), 48–68.

Bryson, A., and MacKerron, G. (2017). Are you happy while you work?, *The Economic Journal*, 127(599), 106–25. doi: 10.1111/ecoj.12269.

Bryson, A., Clark, A. E., Freeman, R. B., and Green, C. P. (2016). Share capitalism and worker wellbeing, *Labour Economics*, 42, 151–8. doi:org/10.1016/j.labeco.2016.09.002.

Bullock, A. (2000). *Building Jerusalem: A portrait of my father*. London: Penguin Books.

Cacioppo, J. T., Cacioppo, S., Gonzaga, G. C., Ogburn, E. L., and VanderWeele, T. J. (2013). Marital satisfaction and break-ups differ across on-line and off-line meeting venues, *Proceedings of the National Academy of Sciences*, 110(25), 10135–40.

Campaign for Dignity in Dying (2015). *Assisted Dying: Setting the record straight*, August. London: Dignity in Dying.

Card, D., Mas, A., Moretti, E., and Saez, E. (2012). Inequality at work: the effect of peer salaries on job satisfaction, *American Economic Review*, 102(6), 2981–3003.

Carlson, M. C., Kuo, J. H., Chuang, Y.-F., Varma, V. R., Harris, G., Albert, M. S., Erickson, K. I., Kramer, A. F., Parisi, J. M., and Xue, Q.-L. (2015). Impact of the Baltimore Experience Corps trial on cortical and hippocampal volumes, *Alzheimer's and Dementia: The Journal of the Alzheimer's Association*, 11(11), 1340–48.

Carneiro, P., Løken, K. V., and Salvanes, K. G. (2015). A flying start? Maternity leave benefits and long-run outcomes of children, *Journal of Political Economy*, 123(2), 365–412.

Case, A., and Deaton, A. (2017). *Mortality and Morbidity in the 21st Century*, Brookings Papers on Economic Activity, Spring, 397.

Chadi, A., Jeworrek, S., and Mertins, V. (2017). Meaningless work threatens job performance, *LSE Business Review*, 19 July.

Chandler, D., and Kapelner, A. (2013). Breaking monotony with meaning: motivation in crowdsourcing markets, *Journal of Economic Behavior and Organization*, 90, 123–33.

Charlson, F. J., Dieleman, J., Singh, L., and Whiteford, H. A. (2017). Donor financing of global mental health, 1995–2015: an assessment of trends, channels, and alignment with the disease burden, *PLOS ONE*, 12(1), e0169384. doi: 10.1371/journal.pone.0169384.

Chilvers, C., Dewey, M., Fielding, K., Gretton, V., Miller, P., Palmer, B., Weller, D., Churchill, R., Williams, I., Bedi, N., Duggan, C., Lee, A., and Glynn Harrison for the Counselling versus Antidepressants in Primary Care Study Group (2001). Antidepressant drugs and generic counselling for treatment of major depression in primary care: randomized trial with patient preference arms, *British Medical Journal*, 322, 1–5.

Clark, A. E. (2001). What really matters in a job? Hedonic measurement using quit data, *Labour Economics*, 8(2), 223–42.

Clark, A. E., Frijters, P., and Shields, M. (2008). Relative income, happiness and utility: an explanation for the Easterlin paradox and other puzzles, *Journal of Economic Literature*, 46(1), 95–144.

Clark, A. E., Lekfuangfu, W., Powdthavee, N., and Ward, G. (2015). *Breaking Up for the Kids' Sake: Evidence from a British birth cohort.* LSE mimeo.

Clark, A. E, Flèche, S., Layard, R., Powdthavee, N., and Ward, G. (2016). *Origins of Happiness: Evidence and policy implications*, VOX CEPR Policy Portal, 12 December.

Clark, A. E., Flèche, S., Layard, R., Powdthavee, N., and Ward, G. (2018). *The Origins of Happiness: The science of well-being over the life course.* Princeton, NJ: Princeton University Press.

Clark, D. M. (2018). Realizing the mass public benefit of evidence-based psychological therapies: the IAPT program, *Annual Review of Clinical Psychology*, 7(14), 159–83.

Clark, D. M., Canvin, L., Green, J., Layard, R., Pilling, S. and Janecka, M. (2018). Transparency about the outcomes of mental health services (IAPT approach): an analysis of public data, *The Lancet*, 391(10121), 679–86.

Clarke, T. C., Black, L. I., Stussman, B. J., Barnes, P. M., and Nahin, R. L. (2015). Trends in the use of complementary health approaches among adults: United States, 2002–2012, *National Health Statistics Reports*, (79), 1–16.

Claxton, K., Martin, S., Soares, M., Rice, N., Spackman, E., Hinde, S., Devlin, N., Smith, P. C., and Sculpher, M. (2015). Methods for the estimation of the National Institute for Health and Care Excellence cost-effectiveness threshold, *Health Technology Assessment*, 19(14), 1–503, v–vi. doi: 10.3310/hta19140.

Cohen, S., and Spacapan, S. (1984). The social psychology of noise, in D. M. Jones and A. J. Chapman, *Noise and Society*. Chichester: John Wiley, pp. 221–45.

Cohn, A., Fehr, E., Herrmann, B., and Schneider, F. (2014). Social comparison and effort provision: evidence from a field experiment, *Journal of the European Economic Association*, 12(4), 877–98. doi: 10.1111/jeea.12079.

Collier, P. (2013). *Exodus: How migration is changing our world.* Oxford: Oxford University Press.

Collier, P. (2018). *The Future of Capitalism: Facing the new anxieties.* London: Penguin Books.

Collins, J. (2001). *Good to Great: Why some companies make the leap . . . and others don't.* London: HarperCollins.

Collishaw, S., Maughan, B., Goodman, R., and Pickles, A. (2004). Time trends in adolescent mental health, *Journal of Child Psychology and Psychiatry*, 45(8), 1350–62. doi: 10.1111/j.1469-7610.2004.00335.x.

Conolly, A., Fuller, E., Jones, H., Maplethorpe, N., Sondaal, A., and Wardle, H. (2017). *Gambling Behaviour in Great Britain in 2015. Evidence from England, Scotland and Wales*. London: National Centre for Social Research.

Council of Economic Advisers (CEA) (2017). *The Underestimated Cost of the Opioid Crisis*. Washington DC: Executive Office of the United States.

Cowan, C. P., Cowan, P. A., Pruett, M. K., and Pruett, K. (2007). An approach to preventing coparenting conflict and divorce in low-income families: strengthening couple relationships and fostering fathers' involvement, *Family Process*, 46(1), 109–21.

Cowan, P., and Cowan, C. (2008). Diverging family policies to promote children's well-being in the UK and US: some relevant data from family research and intervention studies, *Journal of Children's Services*, 3(4), 4–16. doi:10.1108/17466660200800022.

Craig, A., Tran, Y., Hermens, G., Williams, L., Kemp, A., Morris, C., and Gordon, E. (2009). Psychological and neural correlates of emotional intelligence in a large sample of adult males and females, *Personality and Individual Differences*, 46(2), 111–15.

Croson, R., and Gneezy, U. (2009). Gender differences in preferences, *Journal of Economic Literature*, 47(2), 448–74.

Csete, J. (2010). *From the Mountaintops: What the world can learn from drug policy change in Switzerland*, Global Drug Policy Program. New York: Open Society Foundations.

Dahl, M. S., and Pierce, L. (2019). Pay-for-performance and employee mental health: large sample evidence using employee prescription drug usage. *Academy of Management Discoveries*, 26 February.

Dalai Lama (2012). *Beyond Religion: Ethics for a whole world*. London: Ebury Publishing.

Davenport, J., and Tansey, A. (2009). Outcomes of an Incredible Years classroom management programme with teachers from multiple schools. Trinity College Dublin/National Educational Psychological Service; at <http://incredibleyears.com/research-library/>.

Davidson, R. J., and Begley, S. (2012). *The Emotional Life of your Brain*. New York: Hudson Street Press/Penguin Books.

Davidson, R. J., Kabat-Zinn, J., Schumacher, J., Rosenkranz, M., Muller, D., Santorelli, S. F., Urbanowski, F., Harrington, A., Bonus, K., and Sheridan, J. F. (2003). Alterations in brain and immune function produced by mindfulness meditation, *Psychosomatic Medicine*, 65, 564–70. doi: 10.1097/01.PSY.0000077505.67574.E3.

Davies-Cooper, R., Cooper, R., Burton, E., and Cooper, C. L. (2014). *Wellbeing: A complete reference guide*, Vol. II, *Wellbeing and the Environment*. Oxford: Wiley-Blackwell.

de Lazari-Radek, K., and Singer, P. (2017). *Utilitarianism: A very short introduction*. Oxford: Oxford University Press.

De Neve, J.-E. (2018). Work and well-being: A global perspective, in J. Helliwell, R. Layard and J. Sachs (eds.), *Global Happiness Policy Report 2018*. New York: Sustainable Development Solutions Network.

De Neve, J.-E., and Oswald, A. J. (2012). Estimating the influence of life satisfaction and positive affect on later income using sibling fixed-effects, *Proceedings of the National Academy of Science*, 109(49), 19953–8.

De Neve, J.-E., Ward, G., De Keulenaer, F., Van Landeghem, B., Kavetsos, G., and Norton, M. I. (2018). The asymmetric experience of positive and negative economic growth: global evidence using subjective well-being data, *Review of Economics and Statistics*, 100(2), 362–75.

Deacon, B. J., and Abramowitz, J. S. (2005). Patients' perceptions of pharmacological and cognitive-behavioral treatments for anxiety disorders, *Behavior Therapy*, 36, 139–45.

Deci, E. L., and Ryan, R. M. (2012). Motivation, personality, and development within embedded social contexts: an overview of self-determination theory, in R. Ryan (ed.), *The Oxford Handbook of Human Motivation*. Oxford: Oxford University Press, pp. 85–107.

Department of Health and Social Care and Department for Education (2017). *Transforming Children and Young People's Mental Health Provision: A Green Paper*. London: Department of Health; at<https://www.gov.uk/government/uploads/system/uploads/attachment_data/file/664855/Transforming_children_and_young_people_s_mental_health_provision.pdf>.

Deters, F. G., and Mehl, M. R. (2013). Does posting Facebook status updates increase or decrease loneliness? An online social networking experiment, *Social Psychological and Personality Science*, 4(5), 579–86.

Di Tella, R., MacCulloch, R., and Oswald, A. J. (2003). The macroeconomics of happiness, *Review of Economics and Statistics*, 85(4), 809–27.

Diener, E., and Biswas-Diener, R. (2008). *Happiness: Unlocking the mysteries of psychological wealth*. Oxford: Wiley-Blackwell.

Diener, E., and Diener, C. (1995). Factors predicting the subjective well-being of nations, *Journal of Personality and Social Psychology*, 89, 851–64.

Diener, E., Lucas, R., Schimmack, U., and Helliwell, J. (2009). *Well-Being for Public Policy*. Oxford: Oxford University Press.

Dolan, P. (2014). *Happiness by Design: Finding pleasure and purpose in everyday life*. London: Penguin Books.

Domitrovich, C. E., Cortes, R. C., and Greenberg, M. T. (2007). Improving young children's social and emotional competence: a randomized trial of the preschool 'PATHS' curriculum, *The Journal of Primary Prevention*, 28(2), 67–91. doi: 10.1007/s10935–007–0081–0.

Domoslawski, A. (2011). *Drug Policy in Portugal: The benefits of decriminalizing drug use*, report by Open Society Global Drug Policy Program. New York: Open Society Foundations.

Drummond, C., McBride, D., Fear, N., and Fuller, E. (2016). Alcohol dependence, in S. McManus, P. Bebbington, R. Jenkins and T. Brugha (eds), *Mental Health and Wellbeing in England: Adult Psychiatric Morbidity Survey 2014*. University of Leicester: NatCen Social Research and the Department of Health Sciences.

Dryden, J. (1685). *Sylvae* (facsimile). Yorkshire: Scolar Press, 1973.

Duckworth, A. (2016). *Grit: The power of passion and perseverance*. London: Ebury Publishing.

Dunn, E., Aknin, L., and Norton, M. (2008). Spending money on others promotes happiness, *Science*, 319, 1687–8.

Durand, M. (2018). Countries' experiences with well-being and happiness metrics, in J. Helliwell, R. Layard and J. Sachs (eds), *Global Happiness Policy Report 2018*. New York: Sustainable Development Solutions Network.

Durlak, J. A., Weissberg, R. P., Dymnicki, A. B., Taylor, R. D., and Schellinger, K. B. (2011). The impact of enhancing students' social and emotional learning: a meta-analysis of school-based universal interventions, *Child Development*, 82(1), 405–32.

Dustmann, C., and Fasani, F. (2016). The effect of local area crime on mental health, *Economic Journal*, 126(593), 978–1017. doi: 10.1111/ecoj.12205.

Easterlin, R. A. (2010). *Happiness, Growth and the Life Cycle*. Oxford and New York: Oxford University Press.

Easterlin, R. A., Wang, F., and Wang, S. (2017). Growth and happiness in China, 1990–2015, in J. Helliwell, R. Layard and J. Sachs (eds), *World Happiness Report 2017*. New York: Sustainable Development Solutions Network, pp. 48–83.

Economist, The (2017). The new Arab cosmopolitans, 2 November.

Economist, The (2018). 'Frequent flyers of the NHS': the patients who dial 999 dozens of times a year, 3 May.

Edmans, A. (2011). Does the stock market fully value intangibles? Employee satisfaction and equity prices, *Journal of Financial Economics*, 101, 621–40. doi: 10.1016/j.jfineco.2011.03.021.

Edmans, A. (2012). The link between job satisfaction and firm value, with implications for corporate social responsibility. *Academy of Management Perspectives*, 26(4), 1–19.

Edmans, A., Li, L., and Zhang, C. (2017). *Employee Satisfaction, Labor Market Flexibility, and Stock Returns Around the World*, Finance Working Paper No. 433/2014, February. European Corporate Governance Institute.

Ehrenreich, B. (2010). *Smile or Die: How positive thinking fooled America and the world*. London: Granta.

Einon, D. F., Morgan, M. J., and Kibbler, C. C. (1978). Brief periods of socialization and later behavior in the rat, *Developmental Psychobiology: The Journal of the International Society for Developmental Psychobiology*, 11(3), 213–25.

Einstein, A. (1951). *The Need for Ethical Culture*. Albert Einstein Archives, 28-904.Jerusalem: the Hebrew University of Jerusalem.

Eisenberg, M. E., Olson, R. E., Neumark-Sztainer, D., Story, M., and Bearinger, L. H. (2004). Correlations between family meals and psychosocial well-being among adolescents, *Archives of Pediatrics and Adolescent Medicine*, 158(8), 792–6.

Elliott, E. S., and Dweck, C. S. (1988). Goals: an approach to motivation and achievement, *Journal of Personality and Social Psychology*, 54(1), 5.

EMCDDA (European Monitoring Centre for Drugs and Drug Addiction) (2015). Prevalence of problem drug use per 1,000 inhabitants in Europe in 2015, by country [graph], *Statista*, 30 August; at <https://www.statista.com/statistics/597788/problem-drug-use-prevalence-europe-by-country/>.

Epstein, N. B., LaTaillade, J. J., Werlinich, C. A. (2015). Couple therapy for partner aggression, in A. S. Gurman et al. (eds.), *Clinical Handbook of Couple Therapy*, 5th edn. New York: Guilford Press, pp. 389–411.

EUROCONTROL (2006). *Establishment of 'Just Culture' Principles in ATM Safety Data Reporting*, Advisory material/guidance document. Brussels: European Organization for the Safety of Air Navigation.

Falk, A., Becker, A., Dohmen, T., Enke, B., Huffman, D., and Sunde, U. (2018). Global evidence on economic preferences, *The Quarterly Journal of Economics*, 133 (4), 1645–92. doi: 10.1093/qje/qjy013.

Feinberg, M. E., Jones, D. E., Kan, M. L., and Goslin, M. C. (2010). Effects of family foundations on parents and children: 3.5 years after baseline, *Journal of Family Psychology*, 24(5), 532.

Feinstein, L. (2003). Inequality in the early cognitive development of British children in the 1970 cohort, *Economica*, 70, 73–98.

Fischer, M. S., and Baucom, D. H. (2018). Cognitive–behavioral couple-based interventions for relationship distress and psychopathology in J. N. Butcher and J. M. Hooley (eds.), *APA Handbook of Psychopathology*, Vol. 1: *Understanding, Assessing and Treating Adult Mental Disorders*. Washington DC: American Psychological Association, pp. 661–86.

Flavin, P., Pacek, A. C., and Radcliff, B. (2011). State intervention and subjective well-being in advanced industrial democracies, *Politics and Policy*, 39(2), 251–69. doi: doi:10.1111/j.1747–1346.2011.00290.x.

Flèche, S. (2017). *Teacher Quality, Test Scores and Non-cognitive Skills: Evidence from primary school teachers in the UK*, CEP Discussion Paper (CEPDP1472). Centre for Economic Performance, LSE.

Flook, L., Goldberg, S. B., Pinger, L., Bonus, K., and Davidson, R. J. (2013). Mindfulness for teachers: a pilot study to assess effects on stress, burnout, and teaching efficacy, *Mind, Brain, and Education*, 7(3), 182–95.

Ford, T., Collishaw, S., Meltzer, H., and Goodman, R. (2007). A prospective study of childhood psychopathology: independent predictors of change over three years, *Social Psychiatry and Psychiatric Epidemiology*, 42(12), 953–61. doi: 10.1007/s00127–007–0272–2.

Foresight Mental Capital and Wellbeing Project (2008). *Final Project Report – Executive summary*. London: Government Office for Science.

Fowler, J., and Christakis, N. (2008). The dynamic spread of happiness in a large social network: longitudinal analysis over 20 years in the Framingham Heart Study, *British Medical Journal*, 337, a2338. doi:2310.1136/bmj.a2338.

Franks, J., and Mayer, C. (1996). Hostile takeovers and the correction of managerial failure, *Journal of Financial Economics*, 40(1), 163–81.

Fredrickson, B. (2013). *Love 2.0: How our supreme emotion affects everything we feel, think, do, and become*. New York: Avery.

Fredrickson, B. L., and Branigan, C. (2005). Positive emotions broaden the scope of attention and thought–action repertoires, *Cognition and Emotion*, 19(3), 313–32.

French, E. B., McCauley, J., Aragon, M., Bakx, P., Chalkley, M., Chen, S. H., Christensen, B. J., Chuang, H., Côté-Sergent, A., and De Nardi, M. (2017). End-of-life medical spending in last twelve months of life is lower than previously reported, *Health Affairs*, 36(7), 1211–17.

Gardner, F., Leijten, P., Melendez-Torres, G., Landau, S., Harris, V., Mann, J., Beecham, J., Hutchings, J., and Scott, S. (2019). The earlier the better? Individual participant data and traditional meta-analysis of age effects of parenting interventions, *Child Development*, 90(1), 7–19.

Gautier, F. (2008). *The Guru of Joy: Sri Sri Ravi Shankar and the art of living*. Carlsbad, CA: Hay House.

Gawande, A. (2014). *Being Mortal: Medicine and what matters in the end*. London: Profile Books.

Gehl, J. (2011). *Life Between Buildings: Using public space*. Washington DC: Island Press.

Gehl, J., and Gemzøe, L. (2004). *Public Spaces – Public Life*. Copenhagen: Danish Architectural Press.

Gehl, J., and Rogers, R. (2010). *Cities for People*. Washington DC: Island Press.

Gershuny, J., and Halpin, B. (1996). Time use, quality of life, and process benefits, in A. Offer (ed.), *In Pursuit of the Quality of Life*, pp. 188–210. Oxford: Oxford University Press.

Gifford, R. (2007). The consequences of living in high-rise buildings, *Architectural Science Review*, 50(1), 2–17.

Gilbert, B. J., Patel, V., Farmer, P. E., and Lu, C. (2015). Assessing development assistance for mental health in developing countries: 2007–2013, *PLOS Medicine*, 12(6), e1001834. doi: 10.1371/journal.pmed.1001834.

Gilbert, P. (2010). An introduction to compassion focused therapy in cognitive behavior therapy, *International Journal of Cognitive Therapy*, 3(2), 97–112. doi: 10.1521/ijct.2010.3.2.97.

Glaeser, E. L., Laibson, D. I., Scheinkman, J. A., and Soutter, C. L. (2000). Measuring trust, *The Quarterly Journal of Economics*, 115(3), 811–46. doi: 10.1162/003355300554926.

Global Burden of Disease Study (2015). Global, regional, and national age-sex specific all-cause and cause-specific mortality for 240 causes of death, 1990–2013: a systematic analysis for the Global Burden of Disease Study 2013, *The Lancet*, 385(9963), 117–71. doi: 10.1016/S0140-6736(14)61682–2.

Global Commission on Drug Policy (2014). *Taking Control: Pathways to drug policies that work*. Geneva: Global Commission on Drug Policy.

Global Commission on Drug Policy (2017). *The World Drug Perception Problem: Countering prejudices about people who use drugs*. Geneva: Global Commission on Drug Policy.

Goff, L., Helliwell, J. F., and Mayraz, G. (2018). Inequality of subjective well-being as a comprehensive measure of inequality, *Economic Inquiry*, 56(4), 2177–94. doi: doi:10.1111/ecin.12582.

Goleman, D. (1995). *Emotional Intelligence*. New York: Bantam Books.

Goleman, D. (2003). *Healing Emotions: Conversations with the Dalai Lama on mindfulness, emotions, and health*. Boulder, CO: Shambhala.

Goleman, D., and Davidson, R. J. (2017). *Altered Traits: Science reveals how meditation changes your mind, brain, and body.* New York: Avery.

Gottman, J. M. (1994). *What Predicts Divorce? The relationship between marital processes and marital outcomes.* Hillsdale, NJ: Lawrence Erlbaum Associates.

Grant, A. M. (2008). The significance of task significance: job performance effects, relational mechanisms, and boundary conditions, *Journal of Applied Psychology*, 93(1), 108.

Greenberg, M. T., and Abenavoli, R. (2017). Universal interventions: fully exploring their impacts and potential to produce population-level impacts, *Journal of Research on Educational Effectiveness*, 10(1), 40–67.

Greenberg, M. T., Kusche, A. C., Cook, E. T., and Quamma, J. P. (1995). Promoting emotional competence in school-aged children: The effects of the PATHS curriculum, *Development and Psychopathology*, 7 (1), 117–36.

Greenfield, E. A., and Marks, N. F. (2004). Formal volunteering as a protective factor for older adults' psychological well-being, *The Journals of Gerontology, Series B*, 59(5), S258–S264.

Gruber, J. (2004). Is making divorce easier bad for children? The long-run implications of unilateral divorce, *Journal of Labor Economics*, 22(4), 799–833.

Hagen, J. U. (2015). What can aviation teach business about managing errors? *Yale Insights*, 14 September; <https://insights.som.yale.edu/insights/what-can-aviation-teach-business-about-managing-errors>

Haidt, J., and Lukianoff, G. (2018). *The Coddling of the American Mind: How good intentions and bad ideas are setting up a generation for failure.* London: Penguin Books.

Hale, D., Coleman, J., and Layard, R. (2011). *A Model for the Delivery of Evidence-based PSHE (Personal Wellbeing) in Secondary Schools.* CEP Discussion Paper (CEPDP1071), Centre for Economic Performance, LSE.

Hall, P. A. (1999). Social capital in Britain, *British Journal of Political Science*, 29(3), 417–61.

Halpern, D. (1995). *Mental Health and the Built Environment: More than bricks and mortar?* Abingdon, Oxon: Taylor & Francis.

Halpern, D. (2004). *Social Capital.* Cambridge: Polity Press.

Halpern, D. (2010). *The Hidden Wealth of Nations.* Cambridge: Polity Press.

Halpern, D. (2015). *Inside the Nudge Unit: How small changes can make a big difference.* London: W. H. Allen.

Hanh, T. N. (2001). *Anger: Buddhist wisdom for cooling the flames.* London: Rider.

Hanh, T. N. (2008). *The Miracle of Mindfulness: The classic guide to meditation.* London: Rider.

Hanh, T. N., and Weare, K. (2017). *Happy Teachers Change the World: A guide for cultivating mindfulness in education*. Berkeley, CA: Parallax Press.

Hanson, T. L. (1999). Does parental conflict explain why divorce is negatively associated with child welfare? *Social Forces*, 77, 1283–316.

Hare, A. P. (1981). Group size, *American Behavioral Scientist*, 24(5), 695–708.

Harold, G. T., and Sellers, R. (2018). Interparental conflict and youth psychopathology: an evidence review and practice focused update, *Journal of Child Psychology and Psychiatry*, 59(4), 374–402.

Harold, G., Acquah, D., Sellers, R., Chowdry, H., and Feinstein, L. (2016). *What Works to Enhance Inter-Parental Relationships and Improve Outcomes for Children*, DWP Ad Hoc Research Report No. 32. London: Early Intervention Foundation for Department for Work and Pensions.

Harsanyi, J. (1953). Cardinal utility in welfare economics and in the theory of risk-taking, *Journal of Political Economy*, 61, 434.

Harsanyi, J. (1955). Cardinal welfare, individualistic ethics, and interpersonal comparisons of utility, *Journal of Political Economy*, 63, 309.

Haushofer, J., and Shapiro, J. (2016). The short-term impact of unconditional cash transfers to the poor: experimental evidence from Kenya, *The Quarterly Journal of Economics*, 131(4), 1973–2042.

Hawkes, N. (2013). *From My Heart: Transforming lives through values*. Carmarthen, Wales: Crown House Publishing.

Hawkes, N., and Hawkes, J. (2018). *The Inner Curriculum: How to develop wellbeing, resilience and self-leadership*. Woodbridge, Suffolk: John Catt Educational Ltd.

Helliwell, J. F., and Wang, S. (2011). Trust and wellbeing, *International Journal of Wellbeing*, 1(1), 42–78. doi: 10.5502/ijw.v1i1.9.

Helliwell, J. F., and Wang, S. (2012). The state of world happiness, in J. Helliwell, R. Layard and J. Sachs (eds.), *World Happiness Report*, pp. 10–57. New York: The Earth Institute at Columbia University.

Helliwell, J. F., Huang, H., and Wang, S. (2019). Changing World Happiness, in J. Helliwell, R. Layard and J. Sachs (eds.), *World Happiness Report 2019*, pp. 13–44. New York: Sustainable Development Solutions Network.

Helliwell, J. F., Huang, H., Grover, S., and Wang, S. (2018). Empirical linkages between good governance and national well-being, *Journal of Comparative Economics*, 46(4), 1332–46.

Helliwell, J. F., Huang, H., Wang, S., and Shiplett, H. (2018). International migration and world happiness, in J. Helliwell, R. Layard and J. Sachs (eds.), *World Happiness Report 2018*, pp. 13–44. New York: Sustainable Development Solutions Network.

Helliwell, J. F., Aknin, L. B., Shiplett, H., Huang, H., and Wang, S. (2018). Social capital and prosocial behaviour as sources of well-being, in E. Diener, S. Oishi and L. Tay, *Handbook of Well-being*. Salt Lake City, UT: DEF Publishers.

Helliwell, J. F., Layard, R., and Sachs, J. (eds.) (2012). *World Happiness Report*. New York: The Earth Institute at Columbia University.

Helliwell, J. F., Layard, R., and Sachs, J. (eds.) (2016). *World Happiness Report Update 2016*. New York: UN Sustainable Development Solutions Network.

Helliwell, J. F., Layard, R., and Sachs, J. (eds.) (2017). *World Happiness Report 2017*. New York: UN Sustainable Development Solutions Network.

Helliwell, J. F., Layard, R., and Sachs, J. (eds.) (2018). *World Happiness Report 2018*. New York: Sustainable Development Solutions Network.

Helliwell, J. F., Layard, R., and Sachs, J. (eds.) (2019). *World Happiness Report 2019*, New York: Sustainable Development Solutions Network.

Hewison, D., Clulow, C., and Drake, H. (2014). *Couple Therapy for Depression: A clinician's guide to integrative practice*. New York: Oxford University Press, USA.

HM Treasury. (2018). *The Green Book: Appraisal and evaluation in central government*. London: TSO.

Hollon, S. D., Stewart, M. O., and Strunk, D. (2006). Enduring effects for cognitive behavior therapy in the treatment of depression and anxiety, *Annual Review of Psychology*, 57, 285–315.

Holmberg, S., and Rothstein, B. (2011). Dying of corruption, *Health Economics Policy and Law*, 6(4), 529–47.

Holt-Lunstad, J., Smith, T. B., and Layton, J. B. (2010). Social relationships and mortality risk: a meta-analytic review, *PLOS Medicine*, 7(7), e1000316.

Holt-Lunstad, J., Smith, T. B., Baker, M., Harris, T., and Stephenson, D. (2015). Loneliness and social isolation as risk factors for mortality: a meta-analytic review, *Perspectives on Psychological Science*, 10(2), 227–37.

Hsieh, T. (2012). *Delivering Happiness: A path to profits, passion, and purpose*. New York: Grand Central Publishing.

Hughes, C. E., and Stevens, A. (2010). What can we learn from the Portuguese decriminalization of illicit drugs? *The British Journal of Criminology*, 50(6), 999–1022.

Hughes, E. J. (1963). *The Ordeal of Power: A political memoir of the Eisenhower years*. New York: Atheneum Books.

Hulsheger, U. R., Alberts, H. J., Feinholdt, A., and Lang, J. W. (2013). Benefits of mindfulness at work: the role of mindfulness in emotion regulation, emotional exhaustion, and job satisfaction, *Journal of Applied Psychology*, 98(2), 310–25. doi: 10.1037/a0031313.

Humphrey, N., Lendrum, A., and Wigelsworth, M. (2010). *Social and Emotional Aspects of Learning (SEAL) Programme in Secondary Schools: National evaluation*, Research Report DFE–RR049. London: Department for Education.

Humphrey, N., Barlow, A., Wigelsworth, M., Lendrum, A., Pert, K., Joyce, C., Stephens, E., Wo, L., Squires, G., and Woods, K. (2016). A cluster randomized controlled trial of the Promoting Alternative Thinking Strategies (PATHS) curriculum, *Journal of School Psychology*, 58, 73–89.

Hutchings, J., Daley, D., Jones, K., Martin, P., Bywater, T., and Gwyn, R. (2007). Early results from developing and researching the Webster-Stratton Incredible Years Teacher Classroom Management Training Programme in North West Wales, *Journal of Children's Services*, 2(3), 15–26.

IPCC (2018). Masson-Delmotte, V., et al. (eds.), *Global Warming of 1.5°C. An IPCC Special Report on the impacts of global warming of 1.5°C above pre-industrial levels and related global greenhouse gas emission pathways, in the context of strengthening the global response to the threat of climate change, sustainable development, and efforts to eradicate poverty*. Geneva, Switzerland: World Meteorological Organization.

Ipsos (2016). *Yoga in America Study*. Washington DC: Ipsos Public Affairs for Yoga Journal and Yoga Alliance.

Ipsos MORI (2017). *Ipsos Global Trends: Fragmentation, cohesion and uncertainty*. London: Ipsos MORI.

Ishino, T., Kamesaka, A., Murai, T., and Ogaki, M. (2012). Effects of the great East Japan earthquake on subjective well-being, *Journal of Behavioral Economics and Finance*, 5, 269–72. doi: 10.11167/jbef.5.269.

ISI (2017). *Handbook for the Inspection of Schools: Inspection framework*. London: Independent Schools Inspectorate.

Ivlevs, A., and Veliziotis, M. (2018). Local-level immigration and life satisfaction: the EU enlargement experience in England and Wales, *Environment and Planning A: Economy and Space*, 50(1), 175–93.

Jackman, R., Manacorda, M., and Petrongolo, B. (1999). European versus US unemployment: different responses to increased demand for skill? in R. Layard (ed.), *Tackling Unemployment*. Basingstoke and London: Macmillan Press.

Jacob, J. I., Allen, S., Hill, E. J., Mead, N. L., and Ferris, M. (2008). Work interference with dinnertime as a mediator and moderator between work hours and work and family outcomes, *Family and Consumer Sciences Research Journal*, 36(4), 310–27. doi:10.1177/1077727X08316025.

Jacobs, T. L., Epel, E. S., Lin, J., Blackburn, E. H., Wolkowitz, O. M., Bridwell, D. A., Zanesco, A. P., Aichele, S. R., Sahdra, B. K., MacLean, K. A., King,

B. G., Shaver, P. R., Rosenberg, E. L., Ferrer, E., Wallace, B. A., and Saron, C. D. (2011). Intensive meditation training, immune cell telomerase activity, and psychological mediators, *Psychoneuroendocrinology*, 36(5), 664–81. doi: 10.1016/j.psyneuen.2010.09.010.

Jahoda, M. (1982). *Employment and Unemployment: A social-psychological analysis*. Cambridge: Cambridge University Press.

Jefferson, T. (1809). Letter to the Republicans of Washington County, Maryland, 31 March.

Jekielek, S. M. (1998). Parental conflict, marital disruption, and children's emotional well-being, *Social Forces*, 76, 905–36.

Joseph, D. L., and Newman, D. A. (2010). Emotional intelligence: an integrative meta-analysis and cascading model, *Journal of Applied Psychology*, 95(1), 54.

Kabat-Zinn, J. (1990). *Full Catastrophe Living: Using the wisdom of your body and mind to face stress, pain, and illness*. New York: Delacorte Press.

Kahneman, D. (2011). *Thinking, Fast and Slow*. London: Allen Lane.

Kam, C-M., Greenberg, M. T., and Walls, C. T. (2003). Examining the role of implementation quality in school-based prevention using the PATHS curriculum, *Prevention Science*, 4(1), 55–63.

Kay, J. (1998). *The Role of Business in Society*. Paper presented at the Inaugural Lecture, Said Business School, Oxford.

Kazdin, A. E. (2009). *The Kazdin Method for Parenting the Defiant Child: With no pills, no therapy, no contest of wills*. New York: First Mariner Books.

Kellam, S. G., Mackenzie, A. C. L., Brown, C. H., Poduska, J. M., Wang, W., Petras, H., and Wilcox, H. C. (2011). The good behavior game and the future of prevention and treatment, *Addiction Science and Clinical Practice*, 6(1), 73–84.

Kessler, R. C., Berglund, P., Demler, O., Jin, R., Merikangas, K. R., and Walters, E. E. (2005). Lifetime prevalence and age-of-onset distributions of DSM-IV disorders in the National Comorbidity Survey Replication, *Archives of General Psychiatry*, 62(6), 593–602.

Kim-Cohen, J., Caspi, A., Moffitt, T. E., Harrington, H., Milne, B. J., and Poulton, R. (2003). Prior juvenile diagnoses in adults with mental disorder: developmental follow-back of a prospective-longitudinal cohort, *Archives of General Psychiatry*, 60(7), 709–17.

King, D., Browne, J., Layard, R., O'Donnell, G., Rees, M., Stern, N., and Turner, A. (2015). *A Global Apollo Programme to Combat Climate Change*, CEP Report. Centre for Economic Performance, LSE.

King, D., Schrag, D., Dadi, Z., Ye, Q., Ghosh, A. (2015). *Climate Change: A risk assessment* (J. Hynard and T. Rodger (eds.)). Cambridge: Centre for Science and Policy, University of Cambridge.

King, M. A. (2016a). *The End of Alchemy: Money, banking and the future of the global economy*. London: Little, Brown.

King, V. (2016). *10 Keys to Happier Living*. London: Headline.

King, V., Aires, C., Payne, V., and Harper, P. (2018). *50 Ways to Feel Happy: Fun activities and ideas to build your happiness skills*. London: QED Publishing.

Knabe, A., Schöb, R., and Weimann, J. (2017). The subjective well-being of workfare participants: insights from a day reconstruction survey, *Applied Economics*, 49(13), 1311–25. doi: 10.1080/00036846.2016.1217309.

Knight, C., Haslam, S. A., and Haslam, C. (2010). In home or at home? How collective decision making in a new care facility enhances social interaction and wellbeing amongst older adults, *Ageing and Society*, 30(8), 1393–418. doi: 10.1017/S0144686X10000656.

Knight, J., and Gunatilaka, R. (2018). Migration and happiness in China, in J. Helliwell, R. Layard and J. Sachs (eds.), *World Happiness Report 2018*. New York: Sustainable Development Solutions Network.

Kok, B. E., Coffey, K. A., Cohn, M. A., Catalino, L. I., Vacharkulksemsuk, T., Algoe, S. B., Brantley, M., and Fredrickson, B. L. (2013). How positive emotions build physical health: perceived positive social connections account for the upward spiral between positive emotions and vagal tone, *Psychological Science*, 24(7), 1123–32.

Kramer, P. D. (1994). *Listening to Prozac*. London: Penguin Books.

Krekel, C., Kolbe, J., and Wüstemann, H. (2016). The greener, the happier? The effect of urban land use on residential well-being, *Ecological Economics*, 121, 117–27.

Krekel, C., De Neve, J., Fancourt, D., Layard, R. (2020). *A Local Community Intervention that Raises General Aadult Population Mental Wellbeing and Pro-sociality*, CEP Discussion Paper (September). Centre for Economic Performance, LSE.

Kross, E., Verduyn, P., Demiralp, E., Park, J., Lee, D. S., Lin, N., Shablack, H., Jonides, J., and Ybarra, O. (2013). Facebook use predicts declines in subjective well-being in young adults, *PLOS ONE*, 8(8), e69841.

Krueger, A. B. (ed.). (2009). *Measuring the Subjective Well-being of Nations: National accounts of time use and well-being*. Chicago, IL: University of Chicago Press.

Krueger, A. B., Kahneman, D., Schkade, D. A., Schwarz, N., and Stone, A. A. (2009). National time accounting: the currency of life, in Krueger (ed.), *Measuring the Subjective Well-being of Nations: National accounts of time use and well-being*. Chicago, IL: University of Chicago Press, pp. 9–86.

Kruse, D. L., Freeman, R. B., and Blasi, J. R. (2010). *Shared Capitalism at Work: Employee ownership, profit and gain sharing, and broad-based stock options.* Chicago, IL: University of Chicago Press.

Kuo, F. E., and Sullivan, W. C. (2001). Aggression and violence in the inner city: effects of environment via mental fatigue, *Environment and Behavior*, 33(4), 543–71.

Kuyken, W., Weare, K., Ukoumunne, O. C., Vicary, R., Motton, N., Burnett, R., Cullen, C., Hennelly, S., and Huppert, F. (2013). Effectiveness of the Mindfulness in Schools programme: non-randomised controlled feasibility study, *British Journal of Psychiatry*, 203(2), 126–31. doi: 10.1192/bjp. bp.113.126649.

Lane, T. (2017). How does happiness relate to economic behaviour? A review of the literature, *Journal of Behavioral and Experimental Economics*, 68, 62–78.

Langella, M., and Manning, A. (2016). *Diversity and Neighbourhood Satisfaction*, CEP Discussion Paper (CEPDP1459). Centre for Economic Performance, LSE.

Lawlor, B., Golden, J., Paul, G., Walsh, C., Conroy, R., Holfeld, E., and Tobin, M. (2014). *Only the Lonely: A randomized controlled trial of a volunteer visiting programme for older people experiencing loneliness.* Dublin: Age Friendly Ireland.

Layard, R. (1980). Human satisfactions and public policy, *Economic Journal*, 90(360), 737–50.

Layard, R. (2000). Welfare-to-work and the new deal, *World Economics*, 1(2), 29–39.

Layard, R. (2005a). Rethinking public economics: the implications of rivalry and habit, in L. Bruni and P. L. Porta (eds.), *Economics and Happiness: Framing the analysis.* Oxford: Oxford University Press.

Layard, R. (2005b). *Happiness: Lessons from a new science.* London: Allen Lane.

Layard, R. (2006). Happiness and public policy: a challenge to the profession, *Economic Journal*, 116 (510), C24–C33.

Layard, R. (2011). *Happiness: Lessons from a new science*, 2nd edn. London: Penguin Books.

Layard, R. (2018a). *Should Economists Make More Use of Direct Data on Subjective Wellbeing?* Paper presented at the ASSA Annual Meeting 2018, Philadelphia, USA; at <https://www.aeaweb.org/conference/2018/preliminary/ 1205?q=eNqrVipOLS7OzM8LqSxIVbKqhnGVrJQMlWp1BKLi_ OTgRwlHaWS1KJcXAgrJbESKpSZmwphlWWmloOoFxUUX DAFTA1AegsSooGylkq1XDButx4c>

Layard, R. (2018b). Mental illness destroys happiness and is costless to treat, in J. Helliwell, R. Layard and J. Sachs (eds.), *Global Happiness Policy Report*. New York, NY: UN Sustainable Development Solutions Network.

Layard, R., and Clark, D. M. (2014). *Thrive: The power of evidence-based psychological therapies*. London: Allen Lane.

Layard, R., and Mincer, J. (1985). Trends in women's work, education, and family building, *Journal of Labor Economics*, 3(1), Part 2. null. doi: 10.1086/jole.3.1_p2.2534995.

Layard, R., and Nickell, S. J. (2011). *Combating Unemployment*. Oxford and New York: Oxford University Press.

Layard, R., and O'Donnell, G. (2015). How to make policy when happiness is the goal, in Helliwell, Layard and Sachs (eds.), *World Happiness Report 2015*. New York: The Earth Institute at Columbia University.

Layard, R., and Philpott, J. (1991). *Stopping Unemployment*. London: Employment Institute.

Layard, R., and Walters, A. A. (1978). *Microeconomic Theory*. New York: McGraw-Hill.

Layard, R., Clark, A. E., and Senik, C. (2012). The causes of happiness and misery, in Helliwell, Layard and Sachs (eds.), *World Happiness Report*. New York: The Earth Institute, Columbia University, pp. 58–89.

Layard, R., Jackman, R., and Nickell, S. (1994). *The Unemployment Crisis*. Oxford: Oxford University Press.

Layard, R., Mayraz, G., and Nickell, S. J. (2010). Does relative income matter? Are the critics right? in E. Diener, J. Helliwell and D. Kahneman (eds.), *International Differences in Well-Being*. New York: Oxford University Press, pp. 139–65.

Layard, R., Nickell, S., and Jackman, R. (2005). *Unemployment: Macroeconomic performance and the labour market*, 2nd edn. Oxford: Oxford University Press.

Layard, R., Nickell, S. J., and Mayraz, G. (2008). The marginal utility of income, *Journal of Public Economics*, Special Issue: *Happiness and Public Economics*, 92(8–9), 1846–57.

Layard, R., Bailey, L., Coleman, J., and Judge, E. (2018). *Healthy Minds: A four-year course in secondary schools*, report. Centre for Economic Performance, LSE; at <http://www.healthymindsinschools.org/wp-content/uploads/2017/11/HealthyMinds-Pamphlet-181130.pdf>

Layard, R., and Glaister, S. (eds.) (1994). *Cost-Benefit Analysis*. Cambridge: Cambridge University Press.

Lazear, E. P. (2000). Performance pay and productivity, *American Economic Review*, 90(5), 1346–61. doi: 10.1257/aer.90.5.1346.

Leetaru, K. (2011). Culturomics 2.0: Forecasting large-scale human behavior using global news media tone in time and space, *First Monday*, 16(9).

Leong, L. (2010). *The Story of the Singapore Prison Service: From custodians of prisoners to captains of life*, case study presented at the NS6 International Roundtable, Ottawa, Canada, 4–5 May.

Leuven, E., and Løkken, S. A. (2018). Long-term impacts of class size in compulsory school, *Journal of Human Resources*, 3 August, 0217–8574R0212.

Lewis, M. (2010). *The Big Short: Inside the doomsday machine*. New York: W. W. Norton.

Liberini, F., Oswald, A. J., Proto, E., and Redoano, M. (2017). *Was Brexit Caused by the Unhappy and the Old?*, IZA Discussion Paper No. 11059. Bonn: Institute of Labor Economics.

Liberini, F., Redoano, M., and Proto, E. (2017). Happy voters, *Journal of Public Economics*, 146, 41–57.

Little, A. (2016). *The Parents as Partners Programme: An economic appraisal*, A report for The Tavistock Centre for Couple Relationships, London.

Longhi, S. (2014). Cultural diversity and subjective well-being, *IZA Journal of Migration*, 3(1), 13. doi: 10.1186/2193-9039-3-13.

Lordan, G., and McGuire, A. (2018). *Healthy Minds*, Interim Paper. London: Education Endowment Foundation.

Lucas, R. E. (2003). Macroeconomic priorities, *American Economic Review*, 93(1), 1–14.

Lundberg, U., and Cooper, C. L. (2011). *The Science of Occupational Health: Stress, psychobiology and the new world of work*. Oxford: Wiley-Blackwell.

Lyubomirsky, S. (2008). *The How of Happiness: A scientific approach to getting the life you want*. New York: The Penguin Press.

McDaid, D., Park, A.-L., Knapp, M., Wilson, E., Rosen, B., and Beecham, J. (2017). *Commissioning Cost-Effective Services for Promotion of Mental Health and Wellbeing and Prevention of Mental Ill-Health*. London: LSE Personal Social Services Research Unit for Public Health England; at <https://assets.publishing.service.gov.uk/government/uploads/system/uploads/attachment_data/file/640714/Commissioning_effective_mental_health_prevention_report.pdf>

McHugh, R. K., Whitton, S. W., Peckham, A. D., Welge, J.A., and Otto, M. W. (2013). Patient preference for psychological versus pharmacologic treatment of psychiatric disorders: a meta-analytic review, *Journal of Clinical Psychiatry*, 74(6), 595–602.

McIntosh, S., and Morris, D. (2016). *Labour Market Returns to Vocational Qualifications in the Labour Force Survey*, CVER Research Discussion Paper 002. Centre for Vocational Education Research, LSE.

MacKerron, G., and Mourato, S. (2013). Happiness is greater in natural environments, *Global Environmental Change*, 23(5), 992–1000.

Mackie, C., and Stone, A. A. (2013). *Subjective Well-Being: Measuring happiness, suffering, and other dimensions of experience*. Washington DC: National Academies Press.

McManus, S., Bebbington, P., Jenkins, R., and Brugha, T. (2016). *Mental Health and Wellbeing in England: Adult psychiatric morbidity survey 2014*. University of Leicester: NatCen Social Research and the Department of Health Sciences.

Manacorda, M., and Petrongolo, B. (1999). Skill mismatch and unemployment in OECD countries, *Economica*, 66(262), 181–207.

Marcus, S. C., and Olfson, M. (2010). National trends in the treatment for depression from 1998 to 2007, *Archives of General Psychiatry*, 67(12), 1265–73.

Marlow, S., Hillmore, A., and Ainsworth, P. (2012). *Impacts and Costs and Benefits of the Future Jobs Fund*. Cardiff: Department for Work and Pensions.

Marmot, M., Allen, J., Goldblatt, P., Boyce, T., McNeish, D., Grady, M., and Geddes, I. (2010). *Fair Society, Healthy Lives: The Marmot Review*, a strategic review of health inequalities in England post-2010. London: University College London.

Marshall, L. L., and Kidd, R. F. (1981). Good news or bad news first?, *Social Behavior and Personality*, 9(2), 223–6.

Maslow, A. H. (1954). *Motivation and Personality*. New York: Harper.

Mazzucato, M. (2015). *The Entrepreneurial State: Debunking public vs. private sector myths*. London and New York: Anthem Press.

Meacher, M., and Warburton, F. (2015). *Guidance on Drug Policy: Interpreting the UN drug conventions*, All Party Parliamentary Group for Drug Policy Reform, London.

Meier, S., and Stutzer, A. (2008). Is volunteering rewarding in itself? *Economica*, 75(1), 39–59.

Menting, A. T., de Castro, B. O., and Matthys, W. (2013). Effectiveness of the Incredible Years parent training to modify disruptive and prosocial child behavior: a meta-analytic review, *Clinical Psychology Review*, 33(8), 901–13.

Mill, J. S. (1859). *On Liberty*. Boston, MA: Ticknor and Fields.

Moen, P., Kelly, E. L., Fan, W., Lee, S.-R., Almeida, D., Kossek, E. E., and Buxton, O. M. (2016). Does a flexibility/support organizational initiative improve high-tech employees' well-being? Evidence from the work, family, and health network, *American Sociological Review*, 81(1), 134–164. doi: 10.1177/0003122415622391.

Montgomery, C. (2013). *Happy City: Transforming our lives through urban design*. New York: Farrar, Straus and Giroux.

Moynihan, D. P., and Weisman, S. R. (2010). *Daniel Patrick Moynihan: A portrait in letters of an American visionary*. New York: Public Affairs.

Mudde, C. (2007). *Populist Radical Right Parties in Europe*. Cambridge: Cambridge University Press.

Murthy, R. S., and Lakshminarayana, R. (2006). Mental health consequences of war: a brief review of research findings, *World Psychiatry*, 5(1), 25.

Nafstad, H. E., Blakar, R. M., Carlquist, E., Phelps, J. M., and Rand-Hendriksen, K. (2007). Ideology and power: the influence of current neo-liberalism in society, *Journal of Community and Applied Social Psychology*, 17(4), 313–27.

NatCen (2018). *British Social Attitudes: The 35th Report* [Phillips, D., Curtice, J., Phillips, M. and Perry, J. (eds.)]. London: The National Centre for Social Research; at < http://natcen.ac.uk/our-research/research/british-social-attitudes/>

National Academies of Sciences, Engineering and Medicine (2017). *The Health Effects of Cannabis and Cannabinoids: The current state of evidence and recommendations for research*. Washington DC: National Academies Press.

National Family and Parenting Institute (NFPI) (2000). *Teenagers' Attitudes to Parenting: A survey of young people's experiences of being parented, and their views on how to bring up children*, NFPI survey conducted by MORI. London: National Family and Parenting Institute; see <https://www.ipsos.com/ipsos-mori/en-uk/its-official-your-teenager-loves-you>

Niederle, M. (2016). Gender, in J. H. Kagel and A. E. Roth (eds.), *The Handbook of Experimental Economics*, Vol. 2. Princeton, NJ: Princeton University Press, pp. 481–553.

Nijkamp, P., and Poot, J. (2004). Meta-analysis of the effect of fiscal policies on long-run growth, *European Journal of Political Economy*, 20(1), 91–124.

Norris, P. (2003). Is there still a public service ethos? Work values, experience, and job satisfaction among government workers, in J. D. Donahue and J. S. Nye (eds.), *For the People: Public Service in the 21st Century*. Washington DC: Brookings Institution, pp. 72–89.

Nozick, R. (1974). *Anarchy, State, and Utopia*. New York: Basic Books.

Nutt, D. (2012). *Drugs – Without the Hot Air: Minimising the harms of legal and illegal drugs*. Cambridge: UIT Cambridge Ltd.

O'Donnell, G., Deaton, A., Durand, M., Halpern, D., and Layard, R. (2014). *Wellbeing and Policy*. London: Legatum Institute.

OECD (2012). *Sick on the job? Myths and realities about mental health and work*. Paris: OECD Publishing.

OECD (2013). *OECD Guidelines on Measuring Subjective Well-being*. Paris: OECD Publishing.

OECD (2015). *How's Life? 2015: Measuring well-being*. Paris: OECD Publishing.

OECD (2016). *Strategic Orientations of the Secretary-General: For 2016 and beyond*. Meeting of the OECD Council at Ministerial Level Paris, 1–2 June 2016; at <https://www.oecd.org/mcm/documents/strategic-orientations-of-the-secretary-general-2016.pdf>

OECD (2017). *PISA 2015 Results (Volume III): Students' well-being*. Paris: OECD Publishing.

Oesterle, S., Kuklinski, M. R., Hawkins, J. D., Skinner, M. L., Guttmannova, K., and Rhew, I. C. (2018). Long-term effects of the Communities That Care trial on substance use, antisocial behavior, and violence through age 21 years, *American Journal of Public Health*, 108(5), 659–65.

Office for National Statistics (2016). *English Housing Survey: Housing and well-being report 2014*. London: Department for Communities and Local Government (DCLG).

Okbay, A., Baselmans, B. M., De Neve, J.-E., Turley, P., Nivard, M. G., Fontana, M. A., Meddens, S. F. W., Linnér, R. K., Rietveld, C. A., and Derringer, J. (2016). Genetic variants associated with subjective well-being, depressive symptoms, and neuroticism identified through genome-wide analyses, *Nature Genetics*, 48(6), 624.

Olfson, M., Marcus, S. C., Druss, B., Elinson, L., Tanielian, T., and Pincus, H. A. (2002). National trends in the outpatient treatment of depression, *JAMA*, 287(2), 203–9.

O'Neill, O. (2002). *A Question of Trust: The BBC Reith Lectures 2002*. Cambridge: Cambridge University Press.

Oswald, A. J., Proto, E., and Sgroi, D. (2015). Happiness and productivity, *Journal of Labor Economics*, 33, 789–822.

Otake, K., Shimai, S., Tanaka-Matsumi, J., Otsui, K., and Fredrickson, B. L. (2006). Happy people become happier through kindness: a counting kindnesses intervention, *Journal of Happiness Studies*, 7(3), 361–75.

Ott, J. C. (2011). Government and happiness in 130 nations: good governance fosters higher level and more equality of happiness, *Social Indicators Research*, 102(1), 3–22. doi: 10.1007/s11205-010-9719-z.

Palmer, S. (2007). *Toxic Childhood: How the modern world is damaging our children and what we can do about it.* London: Orion.

Palmer, S. (2016). *Upstart: The case for raising the school starting age and providing what the under-sevens really need.* Edinburgh: Floris Books.

Parekh, B. C. (1993). *Jeremy Bentham: Critical assessments.* London: Routledge.

PATHS (2013). *The PATHS® Programme for Schools (UK version)* in Northern Ireland: Executive Summary. Barnardo's Northern Ireland, Belfast.

Paul, G. L. (1966). *Insight vs. Desensitisation in Psychotherapy: An experiment in anxiety reduction.* Stanford, CA: Stanford University Press.

Peasgood, T., Brazier, J., Mukuria, C., and Karimi, M. (2018). Eliciting preference weights for life satisfaction: a feasibility study. Unpublished mimeo.

Perez-Truglia, Ricardo (2019). The effects of income transparency on well-being: evidence from a natural experiment, 23 February; at <SSRN: <https://ssrn.com/abstract=2657808 or http://dx.doi.org/10.2139/ssrn.2657808>.

Perlmutter, J. S., and Mink, J. W. (2006). Deep brain stimulation, *Annual Review of Neuroscience*, 29(1), 229–57. doi: 10.1146/annurev.neuro.29.051605.112824.

Petrides, K., and Furnham, A. (2000). Gender differences in measured and self-estimated trait emotional intelligence, *Sex Roles*, 42(5–6), 449–61.

Pinker, S. (2011). *The Better Angels of Our Nature: The decline of violence in history and its causes.* London: Allen Lane.

Pinker, S. (2018). *Enlightenment Now: The case for reason, science, humanism, and progress.* London: Viking.

Pitkala, K. H., Routasalo, P., Kautiainen, H., and Tilvis, R. S. (2009). Effects of psychosocial group rehabilitation on health, use of health care services, and mortality of older persons suffering from loneliness: a randomized, controlled trial, *Journals of Gerontology, Series A: Biomedical Sciences and Medical Sciences*, 64(7), 792–800.

Plomin, R. (2018). *Blueprint: How DNA makes us who we are.* Cambridge, MA: MIT Press.

Plomin, R., DeFries, J. C., Knopik, V.S., and Neiderhiser, J. M. (eds.) (2013). *Behavioral Genetics.* New York: Worth Publishers.

Putnam, R. D. (2000). *Bowling Alone: The collapse and revival of American community.* New York: Simon and Schuster.

Putnam, R. D. (2007). *E Pluribus Unum*: Diversity and community in the twenty-first century. The 2006 Johan Skytte Prize Lecture, *Scandinavian Political Studies*, 30(2), 137–74. doi: 10.1111/j.1467-9477.2007.00176.x.

Rajan, R. (2019). *The Third Pillar: The revival of community in a polarised world.* London: William Collins.

Rao, G. (2019). Familiarity does *not* breed contempt: Generosity, discrimination and diversity in Delhi schools, *American Economic Review*, 109(3), 774–809.

Rawls, J. (1971). *A Theory of Justice*. Cambridge, MA: Harvard University Press.

Reinke, W. M., Stormont, M., Webster-Stratton, C., Newcomer, L. L., and Herman, K. C. (2012). The Incredible Years teacher classroom management program: using coaching to support generalization to real-world classroom settings, *Psychology in the Schools*, 49(5), 416–28. doi: 10.1002/pits.21608.

Reuter, P., and Trautmann, F. (2009). *A report on Global Illicit Drugs Markets 1998–2007*. Utrecht: Trimbos Institute and RAND for the European Commission.

Ribeaud, D. (2004). Long-term impacts of the Swiss heroin prescription trials on crime of treated heroin users, *Journal of Drug Issues*, 34(1), 163–94. doi:10.1177/002204260403400108.

Ricard, M. (2015). *Altruism: The power of compassion to change yourself and the world*. London: Atlantic Books.

Ricard, M., and Singer, W. (2017). *Beyond the Self: Conversations between Buddhism and neuroscience*. Cambridge, MA: MIT Press.

Richard, L., Gauvin, L., Gosselin, C., and Laforest, S. (2008). Staying connected: neighbourhood correlates of social participation among older adults living in an urban environment in Montreal, Quebec, *Health Promotion International*, 24(1), 46–57.

Roberts, C., Lepps, H., Strang, J., and Singleton, N. (2016). Drug use and dependence, in McManus, Bebbington, Jenkins, and Brugha, *Mental Health and Wellbeing in England: Adult Psychiatric Morbidity Survey 2014*. University of Leicester: NatCen Social Research and the Department of Health Sciences.

Robertson, I., and Cooper, C.L. (2011). *Well-being: Productivity and happiness at work*. London: Palgrave Macmillan.

Rojas, M. (2018). Happiness in Latin America has social foundations, in Helliwell, Layard and Sachs (eds.), *World Happiness Report 2018*. New York: Sustainable Development Solutions Network (SDSN).

Rosenfeld, M. J. (2017). Marriage, choice, and couplehood in the age of the internet, *Sociological Science*, 4, 490–510.

Rosenfeld, M. J., and Thomas, R. J. (2012). Searching for a mate: the rise of the Internet as a social intermediary, *American Sociological Review*, 77(4), 523–47.

Rutter, M., Belsky, J., Brown, G., Dunn, J., D'Onofrio, B., Eekelaar, J., and Witherspoon, S. (2010). *Social Science and Family Policies*. London: British Academy Policy Centre.

Rutter, M., Bishop, D., Pine, D. S., Scott, S., Stevenson, J. S., Taylor, E. A., and Thapar, A. (eds.) (2008). *Rutter's Child and Adolescent Psychiatry*. Oxford: Wiley-Blackwell.

Sacks, D., Stevenson, B., and Wolfers, J. (2010). *Subjective Well-Being, Income, Economic Development and Growth*, Working Paper 16441. Cambridge, MA: National Bureau of Economic Research.

Sadler, K., Vizard, T., Ford, T., Marcheselli, F., Pearce, N., Mandalia, D., Davis, J., Brodie, E., Forbes, N., Goodman, A., Goodman, R., and McManus, S. (2018). *Mental Health of Children and Young People in England, 2017*. Leeds: NHS Digital.

SAMHSA (2018). *Key Substance Use and Mental Health Indicators in the United States: Results from the 2017 National Survey on Drug Use and Health*, Vol. 18–5068. Rockville, MD: Center for Behavioral Health Statistics and Quality, Substance Abuse and Mental Health Services Administration.

Schulz, M. S., Cowan, C. P., and Cowan, P. A. (2006). Promoting healthy beginnings: a randomized controlled trial of a preventive intervention to preserve marital quality during the transition to parenthood, *Journal of Consulting and Clinical Psychology*, 74(1), 20–31. doi: 10.1037/0022-006x.74.1.20.

Schwartz, S. H., and Rubel, T. (2005). Sex differences in value priorities: cross-cultural and multimethod studies, *Journal of Personality and Social Psychology*, 89(6), 1010.

Scott, J., and Clery, E. (2013). Gender roles: an incomplete revolution?, in Park, A., Bryson, C., Clery, E., Curtice, J. and Phillips, M. (eds.) (2013), *British Social Attitudes: The 30th report*, London: The National Centre for Social Research; at www.bsa-30.natcen.ac.uk.

Scott, S., Briskman, J., and O'Connor, T. G. (2014). Early prevention of antisocial personality: long-term follow-up of two randomized controlled trials comparing indicated and selective approaches, *American Journal of Psychiatry*, 171(6). doi: 10.1176/appi.ajp.2014.13050697.

Segal, Z. V., Williams, J. M. G., and Teasdale, J. D. (2013). *Mindfulness-based Cognitive Therapy for Depression*. New York: Guilford Press.

Seldon, A. (2015). *Beyond Happiness: The trap of 'happiness' and how to find deeper meaning and joy*. London: Hodder and Stoughton.

Seldon, A., and Martin, A. E. (2017). *The Positive and Mindful University*, HEPI Occasional Paper 18. Oxford: Higher Education Policy Institute.

Seligman, M. (2002). *Authentic Happiness: Using the new positive psychology to realize your potential for lasting fulfilment*. New York: Free Press.

Seligman, M. E. P. (2011). *Flourish: A visionary new understanding of happiness and well-being*. New York: Free Press.

Seligman, M., and Adler, A. (2018). Positive Education, in Helliwell, Layard and Sachs (eds.), *Global Happiness Policy Report*. New York: UN Sustainable Development Solutions Network.

Sen, A. (1999). *Development as Freedom*. New York: Knopf.

Sen, A. (2009). *The Idea of Justice*. London: Allen Lane.

Sen, A. (2017). *Collective Choice and Social Welfare* (expanded edition). London: Penguin Books.

Shakya, H., and Christakis, N. A. (2017). Association of Facebook use with compromised well-being: a longitudinal study, *American Journal of Epidemiology*, 185(3), 203–11.

Shantideva (AD700). *Bodhicaryavatara* (*The Way of the Bodhisattva*).

Singer, P. (2015). *The Most Good You Can Do: How effective altruism is changing ideas about living ethically*. New Haven, CT: Yale University Press.

Singer, T. (2015). Empathy and the interoceptive cortex, in Ricard and Singer (eds.), *Caring Economics: Conversations on altruism and compassion, between scientists, economists, and the Dalai Lama*. New York: Picador.

Singer, T., and Ricard, M. (eds.) (2015). *Caring Economics: Conversations on altruism and compassion, between scientists, economists, and the Dalai Lama*. New York: Picador.

Singla, D. R., Kohrt, B. A., Murray, L. K., Anand, A., Chorpita, B. F., and Patel, V. (2017). Psychological treatments for the world: lessons from low- and middle-income countries, *Annual Review of Clinical Psychology*, 13, 149–81. doi: 10.1146/annurev-clinpsy-032816-045217.

Singleton, N., Meltzer, H., Gatward, R., with, Coid, J., and Deasy, D. (1998). *Psychiatric Morbidity among Prisoners in England and Wales*. London: Office for National Statistics for the Department of Health.

Steptoe, A., and Lassale, C. (2018). Happiness at older ages, in Clark, Flèche, Layard, Powdthavee, and Ward (2018). *The Origins of Happiness: The science of well-being over the life course*. Princeton, NJ: Princeton University Press, p. 129.

Steptoe, A., and Wardle, J. (2012). Enjoying life and living longer, *Archives of Internal Medicine*, 172(3), 273–5.

Stevenson, B., and Wolfers, J. (2006). Bargaining in the shadow of the law: divorce laws and family distress, *Quarterly Journal of Economics*, 121(1), 267–88.

Stevenson, B., and Wolfers, J. (2008). Economic growth and subjective well-being: reassessing the Easterlin Paradox, *Brookings Papers on Economic Activity*, 1, 1–87.

Stevenson, B., and Wolfers, J. (2010). *Inequality and Subjective Well-being*, NBER Working Paper. Cambridge, MA: National Bureau of Economic Research.

Stiglitz, J. E., Sen, A., Fitoussi, J. P., (2009). *Report by the Commission on the Measurement of Economic Performance and Social Progress* (CMEPSP); at <http://www.stiglitz-sen-fitoussi.fr/documents/rapport_anglais.pdf>

Stringer, B. (2014). Is the Green Belt sustainable?; at <https://barneystringer.wordpress.com/2014/06/17/is-the-green-belt-sustainable/>

Stuart, R. B. (1969). Operant-interpersonal treatment for marital discord, *Journal of Consulting and Clinical Psychology*, 33(6), 675–82. doi: 10.1037/h0028475.

Syed, M. (2015). How to blame less and learn more, *The Guardian*, 2 October; at <https://www.theguardian.com/commentisfree/2015/oct/02/blame-learn-mistakes>

Tan, E. J., Xue, Q.-L., Li, T., Carlson, M. C., and Fried, L. P. (2006). Volunteering: a physical activity intervention for older adults – the experience Corps® program in Baltimore, *Journal of Urban Health*, 83(5), 954–69.

Tay, L., and Diener, E. (2011). Needs and subjective well-being around the world, *Journal of Personality and Social Psychology*, 101(2), 354, 354–65. doi: 10.1037/a0023779.

Tenney., E. R., Poole, J. M., and Diener, E. (2016). Does positivity enhance work performance? Why, when and what we don't know, *Research on Organizational Behaviors*, 36, 27–46.

Testoni, S., and Dolan, P. (2018). *Assessing the relationship between subjective wellbeing and spending time with family in the outdoors* (secondary analysis), What Works Centre for Wellbeing; at <https://whatworkswellbeing.org/product/family-and-outdoor-recreation/>

Thaler, R. H. (2015). *Misbehaving: The making of behavioural economics*. London: Allen Lane.

Thaler, R. H., and Sunstein, C. R. (2008). *Nudge: Improving decisions about health, wealth, and happiness*. New Haven, CT: Yale University Press.

Thomas, J. (2015). *Insights into Loneliness, Older People and Well-being*. London: Office for National Statistics.

Thomas, R., and Dimsdale, N. (2017). A millennium of macroeconomic data [for the UK], dataset. London: Bank of England; at < https://www.bankofengland.co.uk/statistics/research-datasets>

Tromholt, M. (2016). The Facebook experiment: quitting Facebook leads to higher levels of well-being, *Cyberpsychology, Behavior, and Social Networking*, 19(11), 661–6.

Tseloni, A., Mailley, J., Farrell, G., and Tilley, N. (2010). Exploring the international decline in crime rates, *European Journal of Criminology*, 7(5), 375–94.

Twenge, J. M. (2017). *IGen: Why today's super-connected kids are growing up less rebellious, more tolerant, less happy – and completely unprepared for adulthood – and what that means for the rest of us*. New York: Atria Books.

Twenge, J. M., and Campbell, W. K. (2010). *The Narcissism Epidemic: Living in the age of entitlement*. New York: Atria Books.

Twenge, J. M., Gentile, B., DeWall, C. N., Ma, D., Lacefield, K., and Schurtz, D. R. (2010). Birth cohort increases in psychopathology among young Americans, 1938–2007: a cross-temporal meta-analysis of the MMPI, *Clinical Psychology Review*, 30, 145–54. doi: 10.1016/j.cpr.2009.10.005.

UAE (2017). *Happiness Policy Manual*. Abu Dhabi, United Arab Emirates: National Programme for Happiness and Positivity; see <https://www.arabianindustry.com/technology/news/2017/oct/29/uae-launches-worlds-first-happiness-policy-manual-5836714/>

Ulrich, R. S. (1984). View through a window may influence recovery from surgery, *Science*, 224(4647), 420–21.

United Nations Environment Programme (2018). *Emissions Gap Report 2018*. Nairobi: UNEP.

United Nations Office on Drugs and Crime (2005). *World Drug Report 2005*. New York and Geneva: UNODC.

United Nations Office on Drugs and Crime (2016). *Outcome Document of the 2016 United Nations General Assembly Special Session on the World Drug Problem*. Thirtieth Special Session, General Assembly, New York, 19–21 April 2016.

United Nations Office on Drugs and Crime (2018). *World Drug Report Crime Data – Intentional homicide victims*; at<https://dataunodc.un.org/crime/intentional-homicide-victims>

Ura, K., Alkire, S., and Zangmo, T. (2012). Case Study: Bhutan, in Helliwell, Layard and Sachs (eds.), *World Happiness Report*. New York: The Earth Institute, Columbia University.

Urry, H., Nitschke, J., Dolski, I., Jackson, D., Dalton, K., Mueller, C., Rosenkranz, M., Ryff, C., Singer, B., and Davidson, R. (2004). Making a life worth living: neural correlates of well-being, *Psychological Science*, 15(6), 367–72.

Van Rooy, D. L., Alonso, A., and Viswesvaran, C. (2005). Group differences in emotional intelligence scores: theoretical and practical implications, *Personality and Individual Differences*, 38(3), 689–700.

van Schaik, D. J. F., Klijn, A. F. J., van Hout, H. P. J., van Marwijk, H. W. J., Beekman, A. T. F., de Haan, M., and van Dyck, R. (2004). Patients' preferences in the treatment of depressive disorder in primary care, *General Hospital Psychiatry*, 26, 184–9.

Vartanian, O., Navarrete, G., Chatterjee, A., Fich, L. B., Gonzalez-Mora, J. L., Leder, H., Modrono, C., Nadal, M., Rostrup, N., and Skov, M. (2015). Architectural design and the brain: effects of ceiling height and perceived enclosure on beauty judgments and approach-avoidance decisions, *Journal of Environmental Psychology*, 41, 10–18.

Vendrik, M. (2013). Adaptation, anticipation and social interaction in happiness: an integrated error-correction approach, *Journal of Public Economics*, 105, 131–49.

Walker, E., McGee, R. E., and Druss, B. G. (2015). Mortality in mental disorders and global disease burden implications: a systematic review and meta-analysis, *JAMA Psychiatry*, 72(4), 334–41. doi: 10.1001/jamapsychiatry.2014.2502.

Walker, I., and Zhu, Y. (2013). *The Impact of University Degrees on the Lifecycle of Earnings: Some further analysis*, BIS Research paper no. 112. London: Department for Business, Innovation and Skills.

Walsh, L. C., Boehm, J. K., and Lyubomirsky, S. (2018). Does happiness promote career success? Revisiting the evidence, *Journal of Career Assessment*, 26(2), 199–219.

Ward, G. (2015). *Is Happiness a Predictor of Election Results?* CEP Discussion Paper No. 1343. Centre for Economic Performance, LSE.

Ward, G. (2019). Happiness and voting behaviour, in Helliwell, Layard and Sachs (eds.), *World Happiness Report 2019*. New York: Sustainable Development Solutions Network.

Ward, G. (forthcoming). Happiness and voting: evidence from four decades of elections in Europe, *American Journal of Political Science*.

Ward, G., De Neve, J., Ungar, L., and Eichstaedt, J. (2019). (Un)happiness and the 2016 US Presidential Election. Unpublished mimeo.

Webster-Stratton, C., Reid, M. J., and Hammond, M. (2001). Preventing conduct problems, promoting social competence: a parent and teacher training partnership in Head Start, *Journal of Clinical Child Psychology*, 30(3), 283–302.

Webster-Stratton, C., Reinke, W. M., Herman, K. C., and Newcomer, L. L. (2011). The Incredible Years Teacher Classroom Management training: the methods and principles that support fidelity of training delivery, *School Psychology Review*, 40(4), 509–29.

Weinstein, N., Przybylski, A. K., and Ryan, R. M. (2009). Can nature make us more caring? Effects of immersion in nature on intrinsic aspirations and generosity, *Personality and Social Psychology Bulletin*, 35(10), 1315–29. doi: 10.1177/0146167209341649.

West, P., and Sweeting, H. (2003). Fifteen, female and stressed: changing patterns of psychological distress over time, *Journal of Child Psychology and Psychiatry*, 44(3), 399–411.

White, M., Alcock, I., Wheeler, B., and Depledge, M. (2013). Would you be happier living in a greener urban area? A fixed-effects analysis of panel data, *Psychological Science*, 24(6), 920–28.

Whyte, W. H., (1980). *The Social Life of Small Urban Spaces*. New York: Project for Public Spaces.

Wilkinson, R., and Pickett, K. (2008). The problems of relative deprivation: why some societies do better than others, *Social Science and Medicine*, 65(9), 1965–78.

Wilkinson, R., and Pickett, K. (2009). *The Spirit Level: Why equality is better for everyone*. London: Allen Lane.

Wilkinson, R., and Pickett, K. (2018). *The Inner Level: How more equal societies reduce stress, restore sanity and improve everybody's well-being*. London: Allen Lane.

Williams, J. M. G. (2001). *Suicide and Attempted Suicide* (2nd edn). London: Penguin Books.

Williams, J. M. G., and Kabat-Zinn, J. (eds.) (2013). *Mindfulness: Diverse perspectives on its meaning, origins and applications*. London and New York: Routledge.

Williams, J. M. G., and Penman, D. (2011). *Mindfulness: A practical guide to finding peace in a frantic world*. London: Piatkus.

Williams, M. (2014). *Cry of Pain: Understanding suicide and the suicidal mind* (updated and expanded edition). London: Piatkus.

Wilson, B. (2007). *Decency and Disorder: The age of cant, 1789–1837*. London: Faber.

Wolpe, J. (1958). *Psychotherapy Through Reciprocal Inhibition*. Palo Alto, CA: Stanford University Press.

World Economic Forum (WEF) (2012). *Well-being and Global Success*. A report prepared by the World Economic Forum Global Agenda Council on Health and Well-being. Geneva: WEF.

World Health Organization (2009). *Promoting Gender Equality to Prevent Violence against Women*, briefing on violence prevention. Geneva: WHO.

World Health Organization (2017). *Depression and Other Common Mental Disorders: Global health estimates* (No. WHO/MSD/MER/2017.2). Geneva: WHO.

Wu, A. H. (2018). *Gendered Language on the Economics Job Market Rumors Forum*, paper for AEA Papers and Proceedings, 108, 175–9. Nashville, TN: American Economics Association.

Zhang, X., and Oyama, T. (2016). Investigating the health care delivery system in Japan and reviewing the local public hospital reform, *Risk Management and Healthcare Policy*, 9, 21–32. doi: 10.2147/RMHP.S93285.

Picture Credits

Index

80,000 Hours, 97

PELICAN BOOKS

PELICAN BOOKS

PELICAN BOOKS

Social Mobility:
And Its Enemies
Lee Elliot Major and Stephen Machin

National Populism:
The Revolt Against Liberal Democracy
Roger Eatwell and Matthew Goodwin

A Political History of the World
Jonathan Holslag

A Short History of Brexit
From Brentry to Backstop
Kevin O'Rourke

Our Universe:
An Astronomer's Guide
Jo Dunkley

The Art of Statistics:
Learning from Data
David Spiegelhalter

Chinese Thought:
From Confucius to Cook Ding
Roel Sterckx

This is Shakespeare
Emma Smith

What We Really Do All Day
Jonathan Gershuny and Oriel Sullivan

The Government of No One
Ruth Kinna

Plunder of the Commons
Guy Standing